The Care of Wounds

A Guide for Nurses

FOURTH EDITION

Carol Dealey
PhD MA BSc (Hons) RGN RCNT
University Hospital Birmingham
NHS Foundation Trust and University of Birmingham, UK

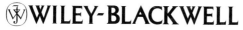
WILEY-BLACKWELL

A John Wiley & Sons, Ltd., Publication

This edition first published 2012 © 2012 by Carol Dealey

Wiley-Blackwell is an imprint of John Wiley & Sons, formed by the merger of Wiley's global Scientific, Technical and Medical business with Blackwell Publishing.

Registered office: John Wiley & Sons, Ltd, The Atrium, Southern Gate, Chichester, West Sussex, PO19 8SQ, UK

Editorial offices: 9600 Garsington Road, Oxford, OX4 2DQ, UK
The Atrium, Southern Gate, Chichester, West Sussex, PO19 8SQ, UK
2121 State Avenue, Ames, Iowa 50014-8300, USA

For details of our global editorial offices, for customer services and for information about how to apply for permission to reuse the copyright material in this book please see our website at www.wiley.com/wiley-blackwell.

Library of Congress Cataloging-in-Publication Data

Dealey, Carol.
   The care of wounds : a guide for nurses / Carol Dealey. – 4th ed.
        p. ; cm.
   Includes bibliographical references and index.
   ISBN-13: 978-1-4051-9569-0 (pbk. : alk. paper)
   ISBN-10: 1-4051-9569-X (pbk. : alk. paper)
   I.   Title.
   [DNLM: 1. Wounds and Injuries–nursing. 2. Wound Healing–physiology. WY
154.2]
   LC classification not assigned
   617.1–dc23
                                                                        2011032157

A catalogue record for this book is available from the British Library.

Set in 9.5/12.5pt Palatino by Thomson Digital, Noida, India
Printed in Singapore by Ho Printing Singapore Pte Ltd

1   2012

Contents

Preface   *vii*

1   The physiology of wound healing   1
    Introduction   1
    Definitions associated with wounds   1
    The structure of the skin   2
    Wound healing   3
    Impaired wound healing   9
    Conclusion   12

2   The management of patients with wounds   15
    Introduction   15
    Physical care   15
    Psychological care   39
    Spiritual care   45

3   General principles of wound management   61
    Introduction   61
    Wound assessment   61
    Managing wounds   77
    Documentation   85
    Evaluating the dressing   86

4   Wound management products   93
    Introduction   93
    The development of dressings through the ages   93
    Traditional techniques   100
    The use of lotions   102
    Clinically effective wound management products   108
    Modern wound management products   110

5   The management of patients with chronic wounds   127
    Introduction   127
    The prevention and management of pressure ulcers   127
    The management of leg ulcers   149
    Diabetic foot ulcers   165
    The management of fungating wounds   170

6   The management of patients with acute wounds   185
     Introduction   185
     The care of surgical wounds   185
     Traumatic wounds   199
     The burn injury   205
     Radiation reactions   216

7   The organisation of wound management   227
     Introduction   227
     Managing wounds in the community   227
     Nurse specialists in wound care   228
     Multiprofessional wound care   229
     Wound healing centres   230
     Conclusions   230

Index   233

Preface

Since writing the previous edition of this book there have been many developments in wound care, especially an increase in the number of guidelines available to healthcare professionals. There is also increasing recognition of the importance of multiprofessional working. The advances in communication mean that we are much more aware of what is happening around the world. I hope that I have reflected some of this in this new edition of *The Care of Wounds* and that this book will be of use to those of you providing care to patients with wounds.

Carol Dealey

1 The Physiology of Wound Healing

Introduction

Wound healing is a highly complex process. It is important that the nurse has an understanding of the physiological processes involved for several reasons:

- understanding the physiology of skin assists in understanding the healing process;
- an understanding of the physiology of wound healing makes it possible to recognise the abnormal;
- recognition of the stages of healing allows the selection of appropriate dressings;
- understanding of the requirements of the healing process means that appropriate nutrition can, as far as is possible, be given to the patient.

Definitions associated with wounds

Any damage leading to a break in the continuity of the skin can be called a wound. There are several causes of wounding:

- traumatic – mechanical, chemical, physical;
- intentional – surgery;
- ischaemia – e.g. arterial leg ulcer;
- pressure – e.g. pressure sore.

In both traumatic and intentional injury there is rupture of the blood vessels, which results in bleeding followed by clot formation. In wounds caused by ischaemia or pressure the blood supply is disrupted by local occlusion of the microcirculation. Tissue necrosis follows and results in ulcer formation, possibly with a necrotic eschar or scab.

The Care of Wounds: A Guide for Nurses, Fourth Edition. Carol Dealey.
© 2012 Carol Dealey. Published 2012 by John Wiley & Sons, Ltd.

Wounds in the skin, or deeper have been labelled in various ways. Some of them can be described as follows.

(1) *Partial- and full-thickness wounds*
  - A partial-thickness wound is one where some of the dermis remains and there are shafts of hair follicles or sweat glands.
  - In a full-thickness wound all the dermis is destroyed and deeper layers may also be involved.
(2) *Healing by first and second intention*
  - These definitions were first described by Hippocrates around 350 BC.
  - Healing by first intention is when there is no tissue loss and the skin edges are held in apposition to each other, such as a sutured wound.
  - Healing by second intention means a wound where there has been tissue loss and the skin edges are far apart, such as a leg ulcer.
(3) *Open and closed wounds*
  - These are the same as healing by second and first intention respectively.

The structure of the skin

The skin is the largest and one of the most active organs of the body. It is composed of two layers: the epidermis and dermis with the epidermis forming the outer surface of the body and the dermis forming the deeper layer of the skin. The main structures of the skin can be found in the dermis. Figure 1.1 shows a cross-section of the skin.

Dermis

Dermis is composed of connective tissue, both collagen and elastic fibres, which is both elastic and resilient and provides support for the structures in the dermis. Blood vessels, lymph vessels, sensory nerve endings, sweat and sebaceous glands and hair follicles can be found within the dermis. The ducts of the glands and hair shafts pass through the epidermis to the skin surface. Sweat glands have their own ducts opening on the skin surface, but sebaceous glands open onto the hair follicles. The base or bulb of hair follicles is sited deep into the dermis. They are lined with epithelial cells and can play a role in the healing of partial-thickness wounds.

The surface of the dermis where it interlocks with the epidermis is irregular with projections of cells called papillae. The base of the dermis is less clearly defined as it blends into subcutaneous tissue, which contains both connective tissue and adipose tissue and helps to anchor the skin to muscle and bone.

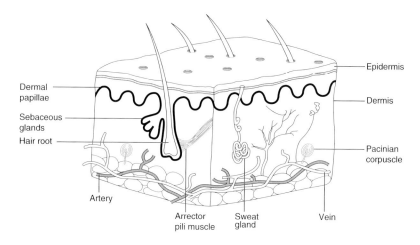

Epidermis

Dermal
papillae

Sebaceous
glands

Hair root

Dermis

Pacinian
corpuscle

Artery

Arrector
pili muscle

Sweat
gland

Vein

Figure 1.1   **A cross-section of the skin**

Epidermis

The epidermis comprises several layers of cells. The deepest layer is the *stratum basale* and it is constantly producing new cells by cell division. These cells are gradually pushed towards the skin surface taking about 7 weeks to reach the surface. The *stratum spinosum* contains bundles of keratin filaments, which hold the skin together. The top three layers of epidermis are the *stratum granulosum*, which produces the precursor to keratin, the *stratum lucidum* and the *stratum corneum.* As they move through the strata, the cells gradually flatten and the protoplasm becomes replaced with keratin. The cells in the *stratum corneum* are flat with no nucleus and are essentially dead cells. They are constantly worn away and replaced by new cells moving to the surface.

In addition the epidermis has cells called melanocytes, which contain melanin that gives skin its colour. A high concentration of melanin produces a dark skin colour. Ultraviolet light increases melanin production. This may occur naturally by sunlight resulting in a suntan or artificially such as a treatment in dermatology.

Wound healing

The wound healing process consists of a series of highly complex interdependent and overlapping stages. These stages have been given a variety of names. They are described here as:

- inflammation;
- reconstruction;

- epithelialisation;
- maturation.

The stages last for variable lengths of time. Any stage may be prolonged because of local factors such as ischaemia or lack of nutrients. The factors that can delay healing are discussed in more detail in Chapter 2.

Inflammation

The inflammatory response is a non-specific local reaction to tissue damage and/or bacterial invasion. It is an important part of the body's defence mechanisms and is an essential stage of the healing process. The signs of inflammation were first described by Celsus, in the first century AD, as redness, heat, pain and swelling. The factors causing them are shown in Table 1.1.

When there is traumatic or intentional injury that causes damage to the blood vessels, the first response is to stop the bleeding. This is achieved by a combination of factors. First, by vasoconstriction that reduces the blood flow and second by the release of a plasma protein called von Willebrand factor from both endothelial cells and platelets, resulting in platelet aggregation and formation of a platelet plug. The third factor is the initiation of the clotting cascade and the development of a fibrin clot to reinforce the platelet plug.

Hageman factor (factor XII in the clotting cascade) triggers both the complement and kinin systems. The complement system consists of plasma proteins, which are inactive precursors. When activated, there is a cascade effect that leads to the release of histamine and serotonin from the mast cells and results in vasodilation and increased capillary permeability. The complement system also assists in attracting neutrophils to the wound. The complement molecule, C3b, acts as an opsonin, that is, it assists in binding neutrophils to bacteria. Five of the proteins activated during the cascade process form the membrane attack complex, which has the ability to directly destroy bacteria.

Table 1.1   **The signs of inflammation**

Signs and symptoms	Physiological rationale
Redness	Vasodilation results in large amount of blood in the area
Heat	Large amount of warm blood and heat energy produced by metabolic reactions
Swelling	Vasodilation and leakage of fluid into the wound area
Pain	May be caused by damage to nerve ends, activation of the kinin system, pressure of fluid in the tissues or the presence of enzymes, such as prostaglandins, which cause chemical irritation

The effect of the complement system is enhanced by the kinin system, which, through a series of steps, activates kininogen to bradykinin. Kinins attract neutrophils to the wound, enhance phagocytosis and stimulate the sensory nerve endings. The apparent delay in feeling pain after injury is explained by the short time lag taken for the kinin system to be activated.

As the capillaries dilate and become more permeable, there is a flow of fluid into the injured tissues. This fluid becomes the 'inflammatory exudate' and contains plasma proteins, antibodies, erythrocytes, leucocytes and platelets. As well as being involved in clot formation, platelets also release fibronectin and growth factors called platelet-derived growth factor (PDGF) and transforming growth factor alpha and beta (TGFα and TGFβ). Their role is to promote cell migration and growth at the wound site.

Growth factors are a subclass of cytokines, proteins that are used for cellular communication (Greenhalgh, 1996). The particular role of growth factors is to stimulate cell proliferation. There are a number of growth factors involved in the healing process, and they are listed in Table 1.2. Some growth factors have been isolated and used as a treatment for chronic wounds. This will be discussed in more detail in Chapter 4.

The first leucocyte to arrive at the wound is the neutrophil. Fibronectin attracts neutrophils to the wound site, a process known as chemotaxis. Neutrophils squeeze through the capillary walls into the tissues by diapedesis, again this ability is enhanced by fibronectin. Within about an hour

Table 1.2 **Growth factors involved in the healing process**

Growth factor	Abbreviation	Action
Platelet-derived growth factor	PDGF	Chemotactic for neutrophils, fibroblasts and, possibly, monocytes. Encourages proliferation of fibroblasts
Transforming growth factor alpha	TGFα	Stimulates angiogenesis
Transforming growth factor beta	TGFβ	Chemotactic for monocytes (macrophages). Encourages angiogenesis. Regulates inflammation
Fibroblast growth factor	FGF	Stimulates fibroblast proliferation and angiogenesis
Epidermal growth factor	EGF	Stimulates the proliferation and migration of epithelial cells
Insulin-like growth factors	IGF-I, IGF-II	Promote protein synthesis and fibroblast proliferation. Work in combination with other growth factors
Vascular endothelial growth factor	VEGF	Critical for angiogenesis and the formation and growth of blood vessels

of the inflammatory response being initiated, neutrophils can be found at the wound site. They arrive in large numbers, their role being to phago-cytose bacteria by engulfing and destroying them. Neutrophils decay after phogocytosis as they are unable to regenerate the enzymes required for this process. As the numbers of bacteria decline, so too, do the numbers of neutrophils.

Transforming growth factor beta attracts monocytes to the wound where they differentiate into macrophages. Fibronectin binds onto the surface receptors on the cells promoting diapedesis and phagacytosis. Oxygen is vital to this process and macrophages can be inactivated and their ability to undertake phagocytosis reduced if the partial oxygen pressure falls below 30 mmHg (Cherry *et al.*, 2000). Macrophages are larger than neutrophils and so are able to phagocytose larger particles, such as necrotic debris, as well as bacteria. The lifespan of the neutrophil can be a few hours or a few days. When they die they are also phagocytosed by the macrophages.

T lymphocytes also migrate into the wound, although in smaller num-bers than macrophages (Martin & Muir, 1990). They influence macrophage phagocytic activity by the production of several macrophage-regulating factors. They also produce colony-stimulating factors that encourage the macrophage to produce a range of enzymes and cytokines. One such substance is prostaglandins, which maintains vasodilation and capillary permeability. It can be produced on demand to prolong the inflammatory response if required. A study by Martin and Muir (1990) found that both macrophages and lymphocytes are present in wounds from day 1, with macrophages peaking between days 3 and 6 and lymphocytes between 8 and 14 days.

Mast cells play a supporting role in the healing process (Ng, 2010). They produce a range of growth factors (PDGF and TGFβ1), inflammatory mediators interleukin 1 (IL-1), tumour necrosing factor alpha (TNFα) and proteases (chymase and tryptase). Chymase and tryptase assist in the breakdown of the extra-cellular matrix in anticipation of the phase of reconstruction.

Inflammation lasts about 4–5 days. It requires both energy and nutri-tional resources. In large wounds the requirements may be considerable. If this stage is prolonged by irritation to the wound, such as infection, foreign body or damage caused by the dressing, it can be debilitating to the patient as well as delaying healing.

Reconstruction

The reconstruction phase is characterised by the development of granula-tion tissue. It consists of a loose extracellular matrix of fibrin, fibrinectin, collagen and hyaluronic acid and other glycosaminoglycans. Macrophages and fibroblasts and the newly formed blood vessels can be found within this matrix. Macrophages play a major role in this phase of healing. They produce PDGF and fibroblast growth factor (FGF), which are both chemo-tactic to fibroblasts, attracting them to the wound and stimulating them to divide and later to produce collagen fibres. Fibronectin has been shown to play a role in enhancing fibroblast activity (Kwon *et al.*, 2007). Collagen has been seen in a new wound as early as the second day. Collagen fibres are made up of chains of amino acids in a triple helix formation. There are a number of different types of collagen characterised by different formations of amino acids. Type III is present in the healing wound in greater proportions than would normally be found in skin. Over time, this pro-portion reduces in favour of higher levels of type I collagen.

Fibroblasts are key cells in this phase of healing (Harding *et al.*, 2002). As well as being responsible for the production of collagen, they also produce the extracellular matrix, which is seen visually as granulation tissue. Tryptase from the mast cells also supports deposition of collagen into the extracellular matrix (Abe *et al.*, 2002). As new extracellular matrix is synthesised, the existing matrix is degraded by enzyme systems such as matrix metalloproteinases (MMPs). There are a number of MMPs, in particular MMP-1, MMP-2 and MMP-9, involved in the healing process, although their role is imperfectly understood at present.

The activity of fibroblasts depends on the local oxygen supply. If the tissues are poorly vascularised the wound will not heal well. The wound surface has a relatively low oxygen tension, encouraging the macrophages to produce TGFβ and FGF, which instigates the process of angiogenesis, the growth of new blood vessels. Undamaged capillaries beneath the wound sprout buds, which grow towards the surface and loop over and back to the capillary. The loops form a network within the wound supplying oxygen and nutrients. Vascular endothelial growth factor (VEGF) produced within the extracellular matrix is responsible for controlling blood vessel forma-tion and growth (Schultz & Wysocki, 2009).

Some fibroblasts have a further role, they are involved in the process of contraction. The exact process is not clearly understood and there are currently two theories postulated: cell contraction and cell traction. The theory of cell contraction is based on specialised fibroblasts known as myofibroblasts and was proposed by Gabbiani *et al.* in 1973. Myofibroblasts have a contractile apparatus, similar to that in smooth muscle cells. In *in vitro* models, they have been shown to cause contraction of the wound. Tomasek *et al.* (1989) found a higher level of contractile forces when a high level of myofibroblasts was present. The concept of cell traction was put forward by Stopak and Harris (1982), who demonstrated that fibroblasts could contract collagen gels by a physical pull, resulting in a rearrangement of the extracellular matrix. Dalton and Ehrlich (2008) reviewed the use of fibroblast-populated collagen lattices to study the process of contraction. As well as myofibroblasts and the concept of tractional forces they describe the mechanism of cell elongation, which also can cause contraction provided there is a high density of fibroblasts. In his review of the role of the mast cell,

Ng (2010) noted that mast cells also seem to be essential for wound contraction. It must be noted that all these studies were undertaken *in vitro* and there is no certainty that they could be repeated *in vivo*.

Whatever the actual process, contraction may start at around the fifth or sixth day. It considerably reduces the surface area of open wounds. Irvin (1987) suggests that contraction could be responsible for as much as 40–80% of the closure. It is certainly of considerable importance in large cavity wounds. However, in shallower wounds with a large surface area such as burns, contraction may lead to contractures. Myofibroblasts disappear after healing is completed.

In wounds healing by first intention, little can be seen of this stage of healing. But in those healing by second intention, the granulation tissue can be seen as it gradually fills the wound cavity. They are followed by capillary buds growing towards the areas of low oxygen tension in the wound.

As the wound fills with new tissue and a capillary network is formed, the numbers of macrophages and fibroblasts gradually reduce. This stage may have started before the inflammation stage is completed and prolonged inflammation can result in excessive granulation with hypertrophic scarring. The length of time needed for reconstruction depends on the type and size of wound, but may be about 24 days for wounds healing by first intention.

Epithelialisation

This phase describes the phase whereby the wound is covered with epithelial cells. Macrophages release epidermal growth factor (EGF), which stimulates both the proliferation and migration of epithelial cells. Keratinocytes at the wound margins and around hair follicle remnants synthesise fibronectin, which forms a temporary matrix along which the cells migrate. The cells move over the wound surface in a leapfrog fashion, the first cell remaining on the wound surface and forming a new basement membrane. When cells meet, either in the centre of the wound, forming islets of cells, or at the margin, they stop. This is known as contact inhibition. Epithelial cells only move over viable tissue and require a moist environment (Winter, 1962). In sutured wounds, epithelial cells also migrate along the suture tracks. They are either pulled out with the sutures, or gradually disappear.

Once the cells stop moving on the wound surface, they start to reconstitute the basement membrane, which is essential in order for the epidermis to 'fix' to the dermis. Until the basement membrane is fully reconstituted it is easy for epithelial cells to be sheared off the wound surface by mechanical forces (Cherry *et al.*, 2000).

Epithelialisation commences as early as the second day in closed wounds. However, in open wounds it is necessary for the wound cavity to be filled with granulation tissue before it can commence. There is a very variable time span for this stage.

Maturation

During maturation the wound becomes less vascularised as there is a reduction in the need to bring cells to the wound site. The collagen fibres are reorganised so that, instead of being laid down in a random fashion, they lie at right angles to the wound margins. During this process, collagen is constantly degraded and new collagen synthesised. The highest level of activity in this process occurs between days 14 and 21 (Cherry *et al.*, 2000). The scar tissue present is gradually remodelled and becomes comparable with normal tissue after a long period of time. The scar gradually flattens to a thin white line. This may take up to a year in closed wounds and very much longer in open wounds.

Tensile strength gradually increases. This is a way of describing the ability of the wound to resist rupture or dehiscence. Forester *et al.* (1969) found that at 10 days an apparently well-healed surgical incision has little strength. During maturation it increases so that by 3 months the tensile strength is 50% that of normal tissue. Further work by Forester *et al.* (1970) compared surgical incisions where the skin edges were held together by tape with those where sutures were used. The findings showed that, when tape was used, the wounds regained 90% strength of normal tissue, whereas sutured wounds only regained 70% strength.

Impaired wound healing

Although the majority of wounds heal without problem, impaired healing may sometimes occur. Some of the different types of impaired healing are described here. Their management will be discussed elsewhere.

Hypertrophic scars

Hypertrophic scars are more common after traumatic injury, especially large burns. They occur shortly after the injury or surgery and remain limited to the area of the injury. They are raised scars with increases in pigmentation, vascularity and pliability (Oliviera *et al.*, 2009). However, they will generally flatten out with time; about 1–2 years.

Van der Veer *et al.* (2009) suggest that an overabundant production of extracellular matrix results in hypertrophic scars that can easily be recognised by their stiffness and rough texture and their colour mismatch. They reviewed all possible activity at the cellular and molecular level to identify any potential causes of this type of scarring and concluded that a number of factors were involved including an increase in the levels of fibronectin, histamine, TGFβ, PDGF, MMPs, IL-4 and IL-13. The impact of this is increased proliferation of fibroblasts and extracellular matrix deposition and reduced collagen breakdown. However, it must be noted that it is still uncertain whether these changes are the cause or effect of scar formation (Van der Veer *et al.*, 2009).

Oliviera *et al.* (2009) compared the levels of types I and III collagen in hypertrophic and normal scars of male children with burns of over 40% of total body surface area. Scars on the thigh following deep burns were studied at 12, 18 and 24 months. Wound biopsies were taken and the collagen levels measured. They found that there was a higher level of accumulation of type III collagen in the deep dermal layer of the skin in the hypertrophic scars when compared with normal scars. There was no difference in type I collagen.

Keloids

Keloids are similar to hypertrophic scars in that they are also the result of an excessive fibrous response. Keloids take some time to form and may occur years after the initial injury. They can range in size from small papules to large pendulous growths (Munro, 1995). Keloids more commonly occur in individuals aged between 10 and 30 years (Cosman *et al.*, 1961) and in those with a darker skin (Placik & Lewis, 1992). Unfortunately, unlike hypertrophic scars, keloids do not gradually flatten out.

Within keloids there are increased levels of collagen and glycosaminoglycan deposition within the extracellular matrix with the collagen presenting as thickened whorls of collagen bundles laid down in a very haphazard manner (Robles *et al.*, 2007). The precise pathogenesis is still unknown, although overexpression of a number of growth factors such as PDGF, TGFα and TGFβ has been identified. In normal healing, there is a negative feedback system to reduce fibroblast proliferation as healing completes. It is proposed that this negative feedback mechanism is deficient in keloidal fibroblasts, allowing scar formation to persist (Robles *et al.*, 2007). Ogawa (2008) has proposed an alternative theory that keloids arise because of a mechanoreceptor or a mechanosensor disorder and that mechanical force or stretching of the skin may be a major causative factor.

Contractures

Wound contraction is part of the normal healing process, but occasionally contraction will continue after re-epithelialisation has occurred resulting in scar contraction (Tredget *et al.*, 1997). Contractures can occur in any wound, but they are more likely if there is delayed healing or in burns (Lee & Clark, 2003). There can be considerable restriction of movement if contractures occur over a joint.

Hildebrand *et al.* (2008) used an animal model to study cellular changes in the presence of contractures and found raised levels of myofibroblasts, TGFβ, MMP-1 and MMP-13 as well as reduced levels tissue inhibitor of metalloproteinases (TIMPs) and changes in collagen structure. The significance of these changes has yet to be ascertained.

Acute to chronic wounds

Chronic wounds may be called chronic because their underlying aetiology makes healing a very long process. A good example is the venous leg ulcer. However, some chronic wounds may have originally been acute wounds that have failed to heal over a long period of time, perhaps years. The original factor delaying healing may have been related to infection or local irritation, perhaps caused by a suture. Once these problems have been resolved the wound still fails to heal causing considerable misery to the patient.

The differences between acute and chronic wounds are still imperfectly understood. However, work by Phillips *et al.* (1998) did shed some light on the problem. They used cultured fibroblasts from human neonatal foreskin as a plated laboratory model and treated them with either chronic wound fluid (CWF) or bovine serum albumen (the control). They found that CWF inhibited the growth of the fibroblasts quite dramatically. The researchers concluded that this study gave some indication of how the microenvironment of a chronic wound has a negative effect on the healing wound. As result of this work, other research groups have looked at wound exudate in more detail.

Trengrove *et al.* (1999) used wound fluid from venous leg ulcers at both non-healing and healing stages to measure MMP levels. They found elevated levels of MMPs at the non-healing stage, which decreased significantly as the ulcers started to heal ($p = 0.01$) The levels of MMPs in the healing ulcers were similar to those in acute wounds, thus suggesting that failure to heal may be linked to excessive matrix degradation. Ladwig *et al.* (2002) collected wound fluid from 56 pressure ulcers and found lower levels of MMP-9 in those ulcers that went on to heal well compared with those that healed poorly.

Trengrove *et al.* (2000) undertook further studies of wound exudate from non-healing and healing leg ulcers. They found significantly higher concentrations of a number of pro-inflammatory cytokines or growth factors in the non-healing ulcers. They consider that wound healing is delayed in chronic wounds because of an impairment of inflammatory mediators rather than any deficit of growth factors.

Subramaniam *et al.* (2008) compared wound fluid from non-healing venous leg ulcers, mastectomy wounds and donor sites to determine MMP levels, TIMPs levels and fibroblast activity. They found a significantly higher level of MMP-1 and MMP-3 production by dermal fibroblasts in the chronic venous leg ulcer fluid compared with the acute wound fluid. There was variation in TIMP-1 levels as the level was very low in both the chronic leg ulcer fluid and the acute graft sites and high in the acute mastectomy fluid. The authors concluded that this could be the result of several variables including the types of wounds and the methods used to collect the wound fluid. Further research s required to obtain greater understanding.

Premature ageing of fibroblasts may also be a problem. Mendez *et al.* (1998) investigated the characteristics of fibroblasts cultured from chronic venous ulcers and found signs of accelerated ageing or senescence in these cells. Senescent fibroblasts have reduced mobility, are less able to replicate, have abnormal protein production and do not respond well to growth factors. A small study of seven patients by Stanley and Osler (2001) compared the senescence rates in fibroblasts taken from chronic venous ulcers with fibroblasts taken from punch biopsies taken from the proximal thigh of the same patient. They found a significantly higher senescence rate in the fibroblasts from the leg ulcers ($p = 0.0001$). Wall *et al.* (2008) found that fibroblasts exposed to chronic wound fluid had a decreased ability to withstand oxidative stress resulting in premature senescence. Telgenhoff and Shroot (2005) suggest this is related to the chronic inflammation found in chronic wounds.

Conclusion

This chapter has described 'normal' physiology. However, not all wounds heal without complication or delay and some of the differences between acute and chronic wound healing have been discussed. But many factors can affect the healing process and they will be considered in more detail in Chapter 2.

References

Abe M, Kurosawa M, Ishikawa O, Miyachi Y (2002) Effect of mast cell-derived mediators and mast cell-related neutral proteases on human dermal fibroblast proliferation and type I collagen production. *Journal of Allergy and Clinical Immunology*, **106**: S78–S84.

Cherry GW, Hughes MA, Ferguson MWJ, Leaper DJ (2000) Wound healing. In: Morris PJ, Wood WC eds. *Oxford Textbook of Surgery*, 2nd edn. Oxford: Oxford University Press.

Cosman B, Crikelair GF, Ju MC, Gaulin JC, Lattes R (1961) The surgical treatment of keloids. *Plastic & Reconstructive Surgery*, **27**: 335–358.

Dalton JC, Ehrlich HP (2008) A review of fibroblast-populated collagen lattices. *Wound Repair & Regeneration*, **16**: 472–479.

Forester JC, Zederfeldt BH, Hunt TK (1969) A bioengineering approach to the healing wound. *Journal of Surgical Research*, **9**: 207.

Forester JC, Zederfeldt BH, Hunt, TK (1970) Tape-closed and sutured wounds: a comparison by tensiometry and scanning electron microscope. *British Journal of Surgery*, **57**: 729.

Gabbiani G, Hajno G, Ryan GB (1973) The fibroblast as a contractile cell: the myofibroblast. In: Kulonen E, Pikkarainen J eds. *The Biology of the Fibroblast*. London: Academic Press.

Greenhalgh D (1996) The role of growth factors in wound healing. *Journal of Trauma*, **41**: 159–167.

Harding KG, Morris HL, Patel GK (2002) Healing chronic wounds. *British Medical Journal*, **324**: 160–163.

Hildebrand KA, Zhang M, Germscheid NM, Wang C, Hart DA (2008) Cellular, matrix, and growth factor components of the joint capsule are modified early in the process of posttraumatic contracture formation in the rabbit model. *Acta Orthopaedia*, **79**: 116–125.

Irvin TT (1987) The principles of wound healing. *Surgery*, **1**: 1112–1115.

Kwon AH, Qiu Z, Hirao Y (2007) Topical application of plasma fibronectin in full-thickness skin wound healing in rats. *Experimental Biology & Medicine* **232**: 935–41.

Ladwig, GP, Robson MC, Liu R, Kuhn MA, Muir DF, Schultz GS (2002) Ratios of activated matrix metalloproteinase-9 to tissue inhibitor of matrix matello-proteinase-1 in wound fluids are inversely correlated with healing in pressure ulcers. *Wound Repair and Regeneration*, **10**: 26.

Lee D, Clark AJE (2003) Wound healing and suture materials. In: Wray D, Stenhouse D, Lee D, Clark AJE eds. *Textbook of General and Oral Surgery*. London: Churchill Livingstone, pp. 10–11.

Martin CW, Muir IFK (1990) The role of lymphocytes in wound healing. *British Journal of Plastic Surgery*, **43**: 655–662.

Mendez MV, Stanley AC, Phillips TH, Murphy M, Menzoian JO, Park HY (1998) Fibroblasts cultured from venous ulcers display cellular characteristics of senescence. *Journal of Vascular Surgery*, **28**: 1040–1050.

Munro KJG (1995) Hypertrophic and keloid scars. *Journal of Wound Care*, **4**: 143–148.

Ng MF (2010) The role of mast cells in wound healing. *International Wound Journal*, **7**: 55–61.

Ogawa R (2008) Keloid and hypertrophic scarring may result from a mechanoreceptor or mechanosensitive nociceptor disorder. *Medical Hypotheses*, **71**: 493–500.

Oliviera GV, Hawkins HK, Chinkes D, Burke A, Luiz A, Tavares P, Ramos-e-Silver M, Albrecht AB, Kitten GT, DN Herndon (2009) Hypertrophic versus non hypertrophic scars compared by immunohistochemistry and laser confocal microscopy: type I and III collagens. *International Wound Journal*, **6**: 445–452.

Phillips TJ, Al-Amoudi HO, Leverkus M, Park H-Y (1998) Effect of chronic wound fluid on fibroblasts. *Journal of Wound Care*, **7**: 527–532.

Placik O, Lewis VL (1992) Immunological associations of keloids. *Surgery, Gynaecology & Obstetrics*, **175**: 185–193.

Robles DT, Moore E, Draznin M, Berg D (2007) Keloids: pathophysiology and management. *Dermatology Online Journal*, **13**: 9 (http://dermatology-s10.cdlib.org/133/reviews/keloid/robles.html).

Schultz GS, Wysocki A (2009) Interactions between extracellular matrix and growth factors in wound healing. *Wound Repair & Regeneration*, **17**: 147–152.

Stanley A, Osler T (2001) Senescence and the healing rates of venous ulcers. *Journal of Vascular Surgery*, **33**: 1206–1210.

Stopak D, Harris AK (1982) Connective tissue morphogenesis by fibroblast traction. 1. Tissue culture observations. *Developments in Biology*, **90**: 383–398.

Subramaniam K, Pech CM, Stacey MC, Wallace HJ (2008) *International Wound Journal*, **5**: 79–86.

Telgenhoff D, Shroot B (2005) Cellular senescence mechanisms in chronic wound healing. *Cell Death and Differentiation*, **12**: 695–698.

Tomasek JJ, Haaksma CJ, Eddy RT (1989) Rapid contraction of collagen lattices by myofibroblasts is dependent upon organised actin microfilaments. *Journal of Cell Biology*, **170**: 3410.

Tredget EE, Nedelec B, Scott PG, Ghahary A (1997) Hypertrophic scars, keloids and contractures. *Surgical Clinics of North America*, **77**: 701–730.

Trengrove MK, Stacey MC, McCauley S, Bennett N, Gibson J, Burslem F, Murphy G, Schultz G (1999) Analysis of the acute and chronic wound environments: the role of proteases and their inhibitors. *Wound Repair and Regeneration*, **7**: 442–452.

Trengrove NJ, Bielefeldt-Ohmann H, Stacey MC (2000) Mitogenic activity and cytokine levels in non-healing and healing chronic leg ulcers. *Wound Repair & Regeneration*, **8**: 13–25.

Van der Veer WM, Bloemen MCT, Ulrich MMW, Molema G, van Zuijlen PP, Middlekoop E, Niessen FB (2009) Potential cellular and molecular causes of hypertrophic scar formation. *Burns*, **35**: 15–29.

Wall IB, Moseley R, Baird DM, Kipling D, Giles P, Laffafian I, Price PE, Thoma DW, Stephens P (2008) Fibroblast dysfunction is a key factor in the non-healing of chronic venous leg ulcers. *Journal of Investigative Dermatology*, **128**: 2526–2540.

Winter GD (1962) Formation of the scab and the rate of epithelialisation of superficial wounds in the skin of the domestic pig. *Nature*, **193**: 293.

2 The Management of Patients with Wounds

Introduction

This chapter looks at the assessment of the patient with a wound and how appropriate care may be planned and evaluated. When caring for patients with wounds of all types it is important to take a holistic approach to their care, considering physical, psychological and spiritual care as they are inextricably linked. There are many factors that can affect the healing process but if they are taken into account when taking a history and assessing the patient it may be possible to mitigate some of the effects. Nursing interventions are not able to resolve every problem, for example, age. Where nursing interventions can be effective, appropriate strategies are suggested.

Physical care

Nutrition

The precise relationship between wound healing and nutrition remains uncertain (Williams & Barbul, 2003). There is increasing evidence that nutritional deficit impairs healing, such as the study by Legendre *et al.* (2008) that compared 41 patients with leg ulcers with 43 controls (dermatology patients without leg ulcers). The research group found a significantly higher incidence of protein deficiency in the leg ulcer group (27% compared with 2% in controls). Protein deficiency was also independently associated with increase in ulcer size at 12 weeks and the occurrence of wound complications. A number of other studies have identified the impact of malnutrition on the healing of surgical wounds, burns and pressure ulcers (Haydock & Hill 1986; Andel *et al.*, 2003; Mathus-Vliegen 2004). The importance of nutrition in relation to pressure ulcer prevention and management is highlighted by the inclusion of the topic in the international guidelines developed by the National Pressure Ulcer Advisory Panel and the European Pressure Ulcer Advisory Panel (NPUAP/EPUAP, 2009).

The Care of Wounds: A Guide for Nurses, Fourth Edition. Carol Dealey.
© 2012 Carol Dealey. Published 2012 by John Wiley & Sons, Ltd.

Malnutrition is a pathological state that results from a relative or absolute deficiency or excess of one or more essential nutrients. As protein or carbohydrates are used in the largest quantities, they are usually the deficient nutrients. This is referred to as protein–energy malnutrition or PEM. In her *Notes on Nursing, What it is and What it is Not*, Florence Nightingale said 'Every careful observer of the sick will agree in this, that thousands of patients are annually starved in the midst of plenty, from want of attention to the ways which alone make it possible for them to take food' (Nightingale, 1859/1974). A century and a half later this statement is still true. A national nutrition screening survey was undertaken in the UK in 2007 in 175 hospitals, 173 care homes and 22 mental health units. A total of 9336 hospital patients were assessed and 28% were found to be malnourished compared with care homes where 30% of the 1610 residents assessed were malnourished and 19% of the 332 adults in mental health units (Russell & Elia, 2007). A review of malnutrition surveys in hospitalised children undertaken over a 10-year period in several different countries (Germany, France, UK and USA) found a prevalence of malnutrition ranging from 6.1 to 14% whereas in Turkey a prevalence of up to 32% was found in two hospitals (Koen *et al.*, 2008).

Overall, malnutrition is seldom recognised in hospital patients although it has a major impact on morbidity and mortality (Pablo *et al.*, 2003). Correia and Waitzberg (2003) undertook multivariate analysis of the impact of malnutrition on adult hospital patients and found mortality increased to 12.4% compared with 4.7% in the well nourished. Hospital costs increased up to 308.9%. The EuroOOPS study monitored the clinical outcomes in 5051 patients across 26 hospitals in 12 countries in Europe and the Middle East. They found that those identified as being at nutritional risk had significantly higher complication rates, length of stay and mortality rates (Sorensen *et al.*, 2008). Older patients are at particular risk of malnutrition. Guigoz *et al.* (2002) identified malnutrition in 20% of hospitalised patients in a survey of more than 10,000 elderly Swiss people in the community, nursing homes and hospitals. Similar results were found in a Spanish study of hospital patients where 18.2% of patients had severe malnutrition (Cereceda *et al.*, 2003).

Nutritional status

The initial causes of malnutrition may be related to debilitating disease, especially of the gastrointestinal tract, old age, poverty or ignorance. Once admitted to hospital, other factors become relevant. An early study by Hamilton Smith (1972) found that patients are starved for up to 12 hours prior to surgery and for varying lengths of time afterwards. Chapman (1996) showed little had changed in over 20 years. She found that patients fasted for periods ranging from 4 to 29 hours. National guidelines in the UK suggest that patients should have a 6-hour fasting period for food, but may have clear fluids up until 2 hours before their operation (Royal College of Nursing (RCN), 2005). A survey of anaesthetists in five northern-European countries found that the majority also followed this guidance (Hannemann *et al.*, 2006). However, its implementation may be far from perfect. A small qualitative study of 15 nurses found that the ritualistic practice of fasting from midnight was so deeply embedded into practice that it was difficult to change it (Woodhouse, 2006). Although such a small study is not necessarily generalisable to all areas, its findings may well resonate with others.

A long period of pre-operative starvation serves to compound the effects of trauma and surgery, both of which cause marked catabolism. Demling (2009) has described how a hypermetabolic–catabolic state can be seen after injury and which, if left uncontrolled can lead to rapid loss of lean body mass (LBM). A LBM loss of 20% will reduce the body's ability to heal and the wound will stop healing altogether with a loss of 30% or more (Demling, 2009). Miller and Btaiche (2009) describe how a negative nitrogen balance results in poor wound healing and delayed patient recovery. Although some patients will return to a normal diet fairly quickly and so redress the balance, others will receive only intravenous fluids. A litre of dextrose 5% contains approximately 150 calories and normal saline does not contain any at all. These fluids obviously do not provide adequate calories to meet the body's requirements.

Burn patients are particularly vulnerable as they have been shown to develop a higher metabolic rate than other critically ill or injured patients (Lee *et al.*, 2005). It may be exacerbated by pre-existing malnutrition. A survey of 123 elderly burn patients found that 61% had pre-existing malnutrition at the time of injury and, compared with well-nourished burn patients in the same age group, they suffered slower healing, a significant increase in infection and an increase in length of stay (Demling, 2005). Adequate nutrition is therefore essential for burn patients, but there is uncertainty as to the optimal time for commencing nutrition therapy. A systematic review by Wasiak *et al.* (2007) compared early enteral support (within 24 hours of injury) with late feeding (after 25 hours of injury). In the five small studies included in the review there appeared to be some promising results for early nutrition, but insufficient evidence to provide clear guidance on the subject. Enhanced enteral nutrition has also been used, for example in a study by Taylor (1999) of 106 burn patients who received enhanced enteral nutrition (50% of energy and nitrogen requirements). There was a significantly greater incidence of infection and length of hospital stay when there was a delay of 24 hours in commencing the enhanced nutrition treatment.

It is the nurses' responsibility to see that their patients have an adequate diet and there has been much discussion of the topic in recent years (Patel & Martin, 2008). Anecdotal evidence has described how patients have their meal times disrupted by medical ward rounds or by being away from the ward undergoing investigations as well as food being placed out of their reach. However, several audits provide more specific information about the causes of inadequate nutritional care. Kondrup *et al.* (2002) conducted a study of 740 randomly selected patients in 3 hospitals in Denmark and assessed their nutritional risk. A total 167 (23%) were found to be at risk and their intake was monitored. Altogether 77 of these patients were in hospital for more than a week and only 25% actually had a minimum of their nutritional requirement met. Analysis of the reasons for this inadequate feeding identified a lack of local guidelines and insufficient nursing knowledge of nutrition. There were also problems with the suitability of the food provided to patients many of whom suffered from loss of appetite. A further study by the same research group questioned 4512 doctors and nurses interested in nutrition from Denmark, Sweden and Norway about their knowledge of nutritional practice (Mowe *et al.*, 2008). The research team found that the respondents lacked sufficient knowledge to be able to adequately screen patients on admission, assess undernourished patients or to be able to initiate nutritional support.

Hamilton *et al.* (2002) audited nutritional provision for elderly patients in community hospitals in the UK. Analysis of the meals provided in a 14-day cycle found they were inadequate for energy, fibre and vitamin D. The portion sizes were small especially the protein element and many patients did not receive the snacks they required. It should also be noted that the patients were positive about many aspects of their meals and the assistance they received from the nurses. Patel and Martin (2008) also addressed the issues around nutrition in elderly patients and studied 100 elderly patients in an inner-city teaching hospital. Altogether 425 assessments were made of these patients and the authors identified that on 285 (67%) occasions these patients were eating inadequately. They found that acute illness, anorexia and oral problems were most common early in the hospital stay. Other problems that they identified were confusion, mood/anxiety disturbances, catering limitations and dysphagia. When compared with well-nourished patients, it was found the malnourished individuals were more likely to have oral problems and anorexia. The authors suggest that detailed assessment of patients would allow nurses to more effectively target the particularly vulnerable patients and ensure they have an improved nutritional intake.

It is important to identify those who are malnourished in order that appropriate steps can be taken to improve their nutritional status. A number of screening tools have been developed and some have been widely validated. One such is the Mini-Nutritional Assessment Tool (MNA), which has been used to assess elderly patients with leg ulceration (Wissing & Unosson, 2001). The first part of the MNA is a screening tool that identifies those who require more detailed assessment. The second part allows the assessor to identify those at risk of malnutrition and those who are actually malnourished, allowing the healthcare professional to develop an appropriate plan of care.

The British Association for Parenteral and Enteral Nutrition (BAPEN) launched the 'MUST' screening tool in 2003 (Elia & Stratton, 2004). It is a five-step tool that has been validated to use with adults of all ages in both hospital and community settings. It allows the assessor to determine if a patient is at low, medium or high risk of malnutrition and provides appropriate management guidelines, depending on whether the patient is in hospital, a care home or the community. The guidance also provides information on how to calculate height for a patient who cannot be measured in the usual way. Further information can be obtained from www.bapen.org.uk.

Hunt (1997) and her colleagues have devised a nutritional assessment tool that considers various factors that can affect nutritional status. It was devised with patients with wounds in mind. Patients are assessed according to their mental condition, weight, appetite, ability to eat, gut function, medical condition including chronic wounds and age. The tool provides a score that indicates whether the patient is nutritionally at risk. Use of a screening tool can be helpful in identifying those less obviously at risk of poor nutritional status than those discussed above.

Nursing interventions

The nutritional needs for each individual varies according to their age, gender, activity and the severity of any illness. If a patient has been assessed as having a reduced nutritional status or falls into a high-risk category, then his nutritional intake should be very carefully monitored. Each patient requires sufficient nutrients to support his basal metabolic rate, his level of activity and the metabolic response to trauma. Patients with heavily exuding wounds, such as fistulae or leg ulcers, may lose large amounts of protein without it being realised. Table 2.1 shows the nutrients required for wound healing and their sources.

The dietician will be able to help in assessing individual needs, so that very specific individualised goals can be set. If a patient is being cared for at home, the carer must also be involved. Many patients will eat better at home, where they can eat what they want, when they want to. Elderly people may have special problems or needs. One problem may be developing disability. The occupational therapist can give guidance on adapting cooking equipment. Another problem may be lack of education as to what constitutes a 'good' diet. Patel and Martin (2008) identified poor dentition or mouth ulcers as common factors in poor nutritional intake. A new set of teeth may be all that is needed to allow an elderly person to maintain an adequate nutritional status.

There are a number of nutrition guidelines available to support clinical practice, for example the European Society for Clinical Nutrition and Metabolism (ESPEN) has produced guidance on managing the patient journey through enteral nutritional care (Howard *et al.*, 2006). Enteral nutrition is the ideal route for nutritional provision and oral nutritional

Table 2.1 **The nutrients required for healing**

Nutrient	RDA*	Food source	Contribution
Carbohydrates	1600–3350 kcals	Wholemeal bread, wholegrain cereals, potatoes, (refined carbohydrates are seen as 'empty' calories)	Energy for leucocyte, macrophage and fibroblast function
Protein	42–84 g	Meat, fish, eggs, cheese, pulses, wholegrain cereals	Immune response, phagocytosis, angiogenesis, fibroblast proliferation, collagen synthesis, wound remodelling
Fats	1–2% kcals	Dairy products, vegetable oil, oily fish, nuts	Provision of energy, formation of new cells
Vitamin A	750 µg	Carrots, spinach, broccoli, apricots, melon	Collagen synthesis and cross-linking, tensile strength of wound
B Complex	3 mg	Meat (especially liver) dairy products, fish	Immune response, collagen cross-linking, tensile strength of wound
Vitamin C	30 mg	fruit and vegetables (but easily lost in cooking)	Collagen synthesis, wound tensile strength, neutrophil function, macrophage migration, immune response
Vitamin E		Vegetable oils, cereals, eggs	Appears to reduce tissue damage from free radical formation
Copper		Shellfish, liver, meat, bread	Collagen synthesis, leucocyte formation
Iron	10–12 mg	Meat (especially offal), eggs, dried fruit	Collagen synthesis, oxygen delivery
Zinc	12–15 mg	Oysters, meat, whole cereals, cheese	Enhances cell proliferation, increases epithelialisation, improves collagen strength

*These recommended daily amounts (RDAs) are the requirements in a healthy individual and may need to be increased (see text).

supplements and tube feeding can be used to supplement patients' diet until such time that they are able to eat normally. The guidelines from the National Institute for Health and Clinical Excellence (NICE) include parenteral as well as enteral nutrition (NICE, 2006). Parenteral nutrition may be used for patients who are unable to tolerate an enteral intake for whatever reason. Nutrients need to be prescribed on an individual basis and should be introduced cautiously for those who are critically ill or seriously injured. Burn patients need very specific management and Prelack *et al.* (2007) have provided practical guidelines for nutritional management not just in the initial stages of injury but also in the recovery phase.

Monitoring outcomes

Evaluation of outcomes may be achieved by regular weighing of the patient and re-assessment using a nutritional screening tool, for example

Gazzotti *et al.* (2003) used weighing and MNA to assess the outcome of a randomised trial to determine the effectiveness of nutritional supplements in preventing malnutrition.

Infection

Consideration of infection must include both systemic and localised wound infection. There is limited knowledge about the precise impact of sepsis on wound healing and what knowledge there is has been mostly gained from animal studies. Rico *et al.* (2002) found that despite infected mice having raised white blood cell and neutrophil counts peripherally, there were significantly lower levels in their wounds. The study team also examined the collagen levels re-epithelialisation rates and found them to be significantly lower in the experimental group compared with controls. Healing may not take place until after the body has dealt with the infection. In addition, systemic infection is frequently associated with pyrexia. Pyrexia causes an increase in the metabolic rate, thus increasing catabolism or tissue breakdown. Infection in a burn wound further increases the metabolic rate and thereby increases the time with a negative nitrogen balance.

All wounds are contaminated with bacteria, especially open wounds. This does not affect healing. However, clinical infection will certainly do so. A review by White *et al.* (2006) suggests several ways in which bacterial virulence factors can have an impact on wound healing:

- bacteria consume the nutrients and oxygen required for wound repair;
- virulent bacteria damage the extracellular matrix;
- anaerobic bacteria impair white cell function;
- oxygen-free radicals increase in numbers and disrupt the balance between matrix metalloproteinases (MMPs) and tissue inhibitor of metalloproteinases (TIMPs);
- the ability of fibroblasts to produce collagen is inhibited and any collagen produced is disorganised.

Recently there has been research into the role of biofilms in wound infection. Biofilms are complex structures that are created when bacteria attach themselves to the wound surface and then surround themselves with a protective polymeric matrix (Bjarnsholt *et al.*, 2008). More than one type of bacteria can be present in a biofilm, including anaerobic bacteria not found by cultures from wound swabs (James *et al.*, 2008). In their study of biofilms in acute and chronic wounds James *et al.* (2008) found them to be present in only 1/16 of acute wounds (6%) in comparison with 30/50 of chronic wounds (60%). Clinical signs of a biofilm infection include an infection that has lasted more than 30 days and seems to wax and wane. It may appear to respond to antibiotics only to recur when the course is completed (Wolcott *et al.*, 2010b). Wound swabs are ineffective in identifying biofilms but molecular diagnositics have been used successfully in specialised centres (Wolcott *et al.*, 2010a).

Some patients are more vulnerable than others to wound infection. Research undertaken looking at surgical wounds has identified a number of factors that increase the risk of developing a wound infection. These studies have been reviewed and then summarised in the *NICE Clinical Guidelines on Surgical Site Infection* (National Collaborating Centre (NCC) for Women's and Children's Health, 2008). They are discussed below.

Age

A review of five studies found age to be a significant independent predictor of the risk of surgical site infection (SSI). The reviewers also found a direct linear trend of increasing risk with increasing age (NCC for Women's and Children's Health, 2008).

Underlying illness

Severity of illness can be measured by using a classification developed by the American Society of Anesthiologists (ASA) that gives a score of one for those deemed normal healthy individuals moving through to a score of six for those declared to be brain-dead whose organs are being removed for donor purposes (ASA, 2002). The reviewers found for studies that indicated that an ASA score of three or above was significantly associated with SSI development (NCC for Women's and Children's Health, 2008). In addition, diabetes has been found as an independent indicator for SSI in a number of studies, for example Olsen *et al.* (2008) undertook a 5-year case–control study of patients undergoing spinal surgery and, using multivariate analysis, they found that diabetes was an independent risk factor for SSI. (See also section on Diabetes mellitus.)

Obesity

Obesity was found to be an independent risk factor ($p = 0.009$) for superficial SSI in a retrospective multivariate analysis of 3174 patients undergoing spinal surgery (Pull ter Gunne & Cohen, 2009). Similarly, a 5-year surveillance programme of 2338 patients undergoing breast surgery for cancer found obesity to be one of the risk factors for SSI (Vilar-Compte *et al.*, 2009). Other studies have found an increased risk of SSI in obese patients in a wide range of surgical procedures including liver transplantation, coronary artery bypass graft and breast reconstruction, (Schaeffer *et al.*, 2009; Russo & Spelman, 2002; Pinsolle *et al.*, 2006).

Nutritional status

Poor nutrition increases the infection risk. A survey of 7035 patients with SSI following general or vascular surgery found that pre-operative albumen levels of $\leq 3.5\,\text{g/dl}$ was an independent risk factor for SSI (Neumayer *et al.*, 2007). (See also section on Nutrition.)

Smoking

Smoking has been shown to cause vasoconstriction (see also section on smoking) and has been identified as an independent risk factor in the review undertaken by for the NICE guidelines (NCC for Women's and Children's Health, 2008). For example, Neumayer *et al.* (2007) in their study of 7035 SSIs found smoking to be an independent risk factor.

Special risks

Irradiation, chemotherapy and steroids, cause greatly increased infection rates and have been identified as independent risk factors by Pinsolle *et al.* (2006), Neumayer *et al.* (2007) and Vilar-Compte *et al.* (2009).

Length of pre-operative stay

The longer anyone is in hospital the more chance there is that the patient's skin becomes colonised by bacteria against which the patient has no resistance. A pre-operative stay over 4 days was found to be an independent risk factor by de Boer *et al.* (1999), Herruzo-Cabrera *et al.* (2004) and Kaya *et al.* (2006).

Shave

It is impossible to carry out a shave without causing injury to the skin. Bacteria flourish and multiply rapidly in these minute cuts. Mishriki *et al.* (1990) and Moro *et al.* (1996) found shaving to be a significant factor in the development of infection. Mishriki *et al.* suggest that this is particularly so when contaminated and dirty procedures are undertaken and bacteria are shed on the skin. It is generally recommended that if a patient needs to be shaved pre-operatively, it should be done just prior to surgery.

Type of surgery

Infection rates are much higher in some types of surgery than others. This is discussed in more detail in Chapter 6. The appearance of infected wounds will be discussed in Chapter 3.

Nursing interventions

The prevention of infection is the responsibility of all healthcare professionals. There are both general and specific measures that can be taken. Most health authorities have infection control policies that provide guidelines both for the prevention of infection and to reduce the risk of cross-infection. The infection control team, especially infection control nurses can give advice and support.

Guidelines are a useful source of information. The *Epic 2: National Evidence-Based Guidelines for Preventing Healthcare-Associated Infections in NHS Hospitals in England* (Pratt *et al.*, 2007) were commissioned by the UK

Department of Health. It is intended that these guidelines are incorporated into local protocols. A major section of the guidelines covers hand hygiene.

The simplest and most effective measure to prevent infection is good hand hygiene, especially as the spread of infection is mostly by people from people. Cross-transmission has been found to be a major factor in infection threats in hospitals (Pratt *et al.*, 2001). Although the focus is on hospitals, good hand hygiene is also required in the community as many of the patients have complex care needs and are vulnerable to infection (Nazarko, 2009).

Following a national prevalence survey of healthcare acquired infections (HCAI) in Ireland, Creedon *et al.* (2008) undertook an observational study of compliance with hand hygiene guidelines in four hospitals. They found that the hospital with the poorest compliance with the guidelines also had a higher prevalence of HCAI in the national survey than the other three. Jenner *et al.* (2006) observed the hand hygiene of 71 healthcare professionals on two medical and two surgical wards and then compared the findings with those of a questionnaire assessing attitudes and self-reported behaviour of the same group of professionals. The results showed that despite there being a high correlation between self-reported behaviour and intention in the questionnaires, the reality of practice was very different with hand hygiene being undertaken on only 100 occasions of the 642 times when it should have occurred. Education can improve compliance with guidelines as demonstrated by Creedon (2006) who found that a compliance rate of 51% increased to 83% following an educational intervention. However, it should be noted that the educational event was supported by the introduction of alcohol hand rub by each patient's bed.

The studies discussed above do not take into consideration the role of the patient in cross-transmission. They also potentially touch hospital equipment and share bathroom and toilet facilities with other patients. Nurses have a responsibility to assist patients with their hand hygiene when necessary. A survey by Burnett (2009) of clinical ward nurses in a teaching hospital found that the majority (99.8% ($n = 442$)) considered patient hand hygiene to be important in preventing the transmission of infection. Their self-reported behaviour did not always reflect this with 57% ($n = 251$) reporting that they 'sometimes' forgot to encourage patients to wash their hands.

The national guidelines (Pratt *et al.*, 2007) state that: 'Hands must be decontaminated immediately before each and every episode of direct patient contact/care and after any activity or contact that potentially results in hands becoming contaminated'. The systematic review underpinning the guidelines did not find good evidence to support the general use of antiseptic hand washing agents over soap and they concluded that choice of the method of decontamination should depend on assessment of: what is appropriate for the episode of care; what is available and what is practicable.

- Hands that are obviously soiled or could be grossly contaminated must be washed in soap and water.
- Hands should be decontaminated between patients or between different care activities for the same patients. An alcohol-based handrub is recommended.
- Hands should be washed with soap and water after several consecutive applications of alcohol handrub.

In addition to hand hygiene, gloves and plastic aprons should be worn when undertaking procedures involving non-intact skin such as wound care (Pratt *et al.*, 2007). Both items should be for single use and removed as soon as the procedure is completed. Ideally hands should be washed with soap and water after removal.

Smoking

There is increasing evidence that smoking has a deleterious effect on the healing wound. One prospective study of 4855 patients undergoing gastrointestinal surgery found that smokers had a 64% higher risk of SSI and an 80% greater risk of wound dehiscence (Sorensen *et al.*, 2005). The same group studied the impact of abstinence from smoking on healing of experimental incisional wounds in healthy individuals. They compared never-smokers with smokers randomised to either continue smoking or abstinence from smoking for a 4-week period. They found a significantly higher incidence of wound infection in the smokers compared with the never-smokers (12% v. 2%, $p < 0.05$). They also found there was a significant reduction in infection in the abstinent smokers compared with continuous smokers (Sorensen *et al.*, 2003).

Manassa *et al.* (2003) undertook a retrospective study of 132 patients undergoing abdominoplasty and compared outcomes for smokers and non-smokers. They found a significantly higher incidence of wound complications for smokers including wound dehiscence (47.9% v. 14.8%, $p < 0.01$). Increased infection and wound breakdown have also been identified in other types of surgery such as cardiac surgery and breast construction and reduction (Bartsch *et al.*, 2007; Booi *et al.*, 2007; Steingrimsson *et al.*, 2009).

An *in-vitro* study by Ejaz *et al.* (2009) found cigarette smoke condensate severely disrupted angiogenesis and there was deterioration of the extracellular matrix. Sorensen *et al.* (2009) found a two-fold higher level of MMP-8 in wound fluid of smokers compared with never smokers; MMP-8 is a neutrophil collagenase and contributes to increased collagen degradation. The research team also found delayed epidermal healing and an altered inflammatory response.

A more recent study by Sorensen *et al.* (2010) used a similar methodology for 78 healthy volunteers who received repeated punch biopsies at weeks 1, 4, 8 and 12 of a 13-week study. The researchers found that inflammation was initially impaired among the smokers, but for the smokers who were randomised to abstinence the level of inflammation rose to the same level as the never-smokers after 4 weeks. However, abstinence did not reverse the reduction in fibroblast activity and inhibition of collagen production. They conclude that it is possible to reduce the incidence of wound infection with pre-operative smoking cessation and their findings explain why cessation does not reduce the incidence of wound dehiscence.

Smoking may also act as an appetite depressant. Smokers have been found to be deficient in vitamins B_1, B_6, B_{12} and C. Smoking reduces subcutaneous oxygen tension significantly for up to 30–45 minutes after each cigarette. However, most studies in this area have been undertaken looking at surgical wounds and there is little information regarding smoking and chronic wound healing (Sorensen, 2003).

Nursing interventions

Nurses can play a significant role in both educating patients in the harmful effects of smoking on a healing wound and encouraging them to abstain over the peri-operative period. Prescription of nicotine patches may also be helpful for some patients. Additional support from help-lines and other agencies may also be beneficial.

Diabetes mellitus

Both type 1 and type 2 diabetes have been shown to be associated with delayed healing and also a higher level of infection compared with the general population (Patel, 2008). King (2001) suggested infection occurs because high glucose levels encourage proliferation of bacteria. There are, however, a number of other problems that may be encountered in people with diabetes with deep wounds such as surgical incisions. They may be encountered through each stage of the healing process.

- Signs of inflammation may be limited because of a thickened basement membrane causes a rigidity that prevents vasodilation (Renwick *et al.*, 1998).
- In addition, high glucose levels make erythrocytes, platelets and leucocytes more adhesive and they tend to stick together filling the vascular lumen (Alberti & Press, 1992).
- There is decreased phagocytosis and poor chemotactic response in neutrophils that Ochoa *et al.* (2007) suggest is because of alterations in the chemokine system.
- Chbinou and Frenette (2004) found reduced levels of neutrophils, macrophages and angiogenesis in a diabetic animal model
- Several studies have demonstrated that diabetics have abnormal fibroblasts with reduced capacity for proliferation and collagen synthesis.

This results in abnormal cross-linking of collagen and reduced wound contraction, further prolonging the healing process (Loughlin & Arlett, 2009).

- An *in vitro* study found that MMP-2 and MMP-9 were both down-regulated in hyperglycaemic conditions, which the research team believed to be linked to reduced keratinocyte activity resulting in reduced migration and proliferation and inadequate re-epithelialisation (Lan *et al.*, 2008).

- Also, people with diabetes deal with the stress of wounding (trauma or surgery) by producing increased levels of glucagons, cortisol and growth hormone leading to raised levels of blood glucose and an increased need for insulin. If this situation is not corrected the patient can become catabolic. Left untreated, the body will start to break down proteins and fats, ultimately resulting in a state of negative nitrogen balance (Rosenberg, 1990).

Nursing interventions

In planned procedures it is possible to ensure that the patient is adequately prepared and the diabetes well controlled. Obviously this is not possible when a patient suffers traumatic injury. In either event during any period of fasting the greatest risk is from hypoglycaemia and it may be necessary to commence a dextrose intravenous infusion. In the immediate post-operative or post-injury period the patient is at considerable risk of hyperglycaemia as a result of the stress of the event. Perkins (2004) discussed this problem in relation to critically ill patients, in particular the danger of intensive insulin therapy resulting in hypoglycaemia. She proposed that effective interventions could only be achieved by effective multiprofessional teamwork and agreement of planned actions or protocols. Such an agreement would need to consider the frequency of monitoring for blood glucose and the level at which insulin therapy would be commenced. Perkins describes the regime that was set for the critically ill trauma patient: 2-hourly monitoring with insulin therapy set to commence if blood glucose levels rose above 7 mmol/l. Insulin was to be administered according to a sliding scale in order to ensure titration. American guidelines suggest the use of an insulin intravenous infusion is in order to provide tight glucose control (Patel, 2008). Obviously, this level of intervention is not necessary or appropriate for every patient, but the principle of team working and developing agreed planned action can be applied to any situation where diabetic control is challenged because of stress.

The physical effects of stress

Stress has a physiological effect. Stimulated by the release of adrenalin, a primary biochemical change in stress is an increased secretion of adrenocorticotrophic hormone (ACTH), which stimulates production of adrenal cortex hormones. In particular, ACTH regulates production of glucocorticoids, cortisol and hydrocortisone. Glucocorticoids cause the breakdown of body stores to glucose, raising blood sugar. They cause a reduction in the mobility of granulocytes and macrophages, impeding their migration to the wound. In effect this suppresses the immune system and reduces the inflammatory response. Glucocorticoids also increase protein breakdown and nitrogen excretion, which inhibits the regeneration of endothelial cells and delays collagen synthesis.

Kiecolt-Glaser and colleagues (2005) studied 42 healthy married couples who were given suction blister wounds and then assessed for healing following either a social interaction or a discussion resulting in conflict. They found that the wounds healed more slowly after the conflict discussions that the social interaction. The researchers also found that there were higher levels of the pro-inflammatory cytokines interleukin-6 (IL-6) and tumour necrosing factor alpha (TNFα) in the wound fluid following conflict suggesting that stress prolongs inflammation (Kiecolt-Glaser *et al.*, 2005). There also seems to be an increased risk of wound infection in a stressed patient (Kiecolt-Glaser *et al.*, 2002). An animal model study found a significantly higher incidence of opportunistic infection compared with the control group as well a 30% rate of delayed healing (Rojas *et al.*, 2002). Jones *et al.* (2006) assessed 190 patients with chronic venous leg ulcers for anxiety and depression and found that high scores for anxiety or depression were most commonly associated with pain and malodour. A great number of factors can cause stress and they will be discussed throughout the rest of this chapter.

Pain

Pain and stress are closely related because pain can increase stress and stress increase pain (Augustin & Maier, 2003). Fear of pain can cause much anxiety to patients. Pracek *et al.* (1995) found that procedural pain experienced by burn patients in the early stages of their admission could be a causal factor in their ability to adjust after discharge. The greater the pain levels, the poorer the adjustment. Soon and Acton (2006) suggested that persistent wound pain is not only distressing but will ultimately result in psychological problems.

Vuolo (2009) described three types of wound pain: nociceptive, neuropathic and emotional. Nociceptive pain occurs as a result of tissue damage and it can be persistent and may be described as gnawing or aching with tenderness (Coutts *et al.*, 2008). Neuropathic pain is caused by nerve injury and patients may use words such as stabbing, burning, stinging or shooting sensation to describe it (Coutts *et al.*, 2008). Emotional pain may occur because of the psychological impact of the wound maybe because of the impact on body image or physical problems because of odour or leaking exudate (Vuolo, 2009).

There has been increasing recognition of the effect of pain on patients with chronic wounds. Günes (2008) studied 47 patients with pressure ulcers and found that 44 (94.6%) had pain from their ulcer. Those with more severe pressure ulcers described their pain as 'horrible'. Basic activities such as walking, standing or climbing stairs can increase chronic wound pain (Woo & Sibbald, 2008). A large international survey of 2018 patients with chronic wounds was undertaken across 15 countries and found that 31.1% had pain 'quite often' and 36.6% had pain 'most' or 'all of the time' (Price *et al.*, 2008). The survey also addressed pain intensity and found that patients with leg ulcers or burns had the greatest pain intensity. The authors found that 64% of the patients surveyed were taking medication for their pain and of these, 82% found it effective, which they noted to be higher than that found in previous studies (Price *et al.*, 2008).

A small study of women undergoing gastric bypass surgery found evidence of an association between pain and delayed wound healing. Seventeen women were studied for 5 weeks for post-operative pain intensity and subsequent healing of a punch biopsy wound. The researchers found a significant association between greater wound pain and delayed healing of the punch biopsy (McGuire *et al.*, 2006).

Procedural pain such as pain caused by dressing change can be very stressful for patients. Apart from the actual pain caused by the procedure, they may become stressed and anxious anticipating the pain (Woo & Sibbald, 2008). In the survey by Price *et al.* (2008) 40.3% said that pain at dressing changes was the worst part of living with an ulcer.

There is a wealth of evidence that lack of adequate pain control is common. A recent paper by Macpherson and Aarons (2009) examined barriers to effective pain relief in the Caribbean and concluded that they were similar to those found elsewhere in the world namely:

* patient and family attitudes;
* inadequate knowledge or care provision by healthcare professionals;
* organisational factors.

Patient and family attitudes

Many older patients see pain as something that happens as they get older and that they should just live with it. There is also a fear among all age groups of becoming addicted to analgesia (Bell & Duffy, 2009). In addition, many patients may be passive recipients of pain relief, in other words they wait to be asked if they have pain. Manias *et al.* (2006) observed patients' decision-making strategies for managing their post-operative pain and found that this passive approach included waiting to be asked, refusing analgesia even when in pain and postponing analgesia until later. It was the most frequent strategy employed by patients and was more than twice as common as problem-solving with the nurse to plan pain control. The least common strategy was active negotiation by the patient to ask for pain relief and to select one of the solutions proposed by the nurse.

Inadequate knowledge or care provision by healthcare professionals

Macpherson and Aarons (2009) suggest that nurses and other healthcare professionals have inadequate education about pain management. Although this may be true to a varying extent in different countries, nurses' attitudes also need to be taken into consideration. In their review, Bell and Duffy (2009) identified several barriers to effective pain relief raised by nurses: they were too busy; too concerned with the task in hand; they believed that patients should expect pain and often underestimated the level of pain. Dihle *et al.* (2006) undertook observations in surgical wards and conducted in-depth interviews with some of the nurses and found considerable discrepancy between what the nurses said they did and what they actually did. They found that the nurses had theoretical knowledge, but did not always seem to translate it into the clinical setting. Both Dihle *et al.* (2006) and Manias *et al.* (2006) found there was limited use of pain scales despite the considerable amount of research that has been undertaken demonstrating their usefulness. Dihle *et al.* (2006) also noted that very little re-assessment of patients took place following analgesia to determine its effectiveness. This finding is supported by an observational study by Bucknall *et al.* (2007) that set out to determine when and how nurses re-assessed post-operative pain after analgesia. They concluded that there was an extraordinary lack of re-assessment undertaken by nurses.

Organisation factors

Bell and Duffy (2009) suggest that time management is a major barrier to effective pain management. Nurses are constantly interrupted by telephone calls, assisting doctors, dealing with patient admissions and discharges and searching for equipment (Manias *et al.*, 2006). Even when nurses were acting to manage pain effectively, there could be delays because medication needed to be prescribed by a doctor or obtained from the pharmacy.

Parsons (1992) gave an overview of studies of cultural aspects of pain and concluded that definitions of pain by both the sufferer and carer are shaped by cultural beliefs. In some cultures free expression of feelings of pain is expected whereas in others it is unacceptable. There needs to be recognition of these cultural differences in order to manage pain successfully.

Effective pain management

Coutts *et al.* (2008) described the ABCD guide for the management of wound pain:

A = assess the pain;
B = be aware of the cause;
C = consider local treatment;
D = do we need systemic treatment?

A: assess the pain

Pain is very personal and the only person who truly understands it is the patient. Woo *et al.* (2008) suggest that it is best to assume that all patients with chronic wounds have pain unless they indicate otherwise. Coutts *et al.* (2008) suggested it is useful to ask the patient how much the pain has an impact on everyday life such as its impact on sleep, mobility or appetite. It is also useful to know how long the pain has been present and if it is present continuously and, if not, when it starts. The Royal College of Physicians has provided a useful algorithm on assessment in their guidance on assessing pain in older people including those with cognitive impairment (Royal College of Physicians, 2007).

Other information that is needed as part of the pain assessment is to understand the level of pain intensity and what words the patient uses to describe the pain. A number of scales have been developed to assess pain intensity. Most of them involve a numerical rating where the highest score is the worst pain imaginable and the lowest (usually zero) is no pain. Figure 2.1 shows a pain scale that also includes a list of words to assist patients in selecting the best descriptor for their pain. Where patients are unable to communicate with staff about their pain other methods of assessment are required. This might include observing facial expressions and body movements (Royal College of Physicians, 2007). Li *et al.* (2008) reviewed assessment tools available to patients in critical care. They concluded that the Behavioural Pain Scale and the Critical-Care Pain Observation Tool showed validity and reliability but there was a need for a more rigorous evaluation to determine their robustness.

In the Wound Pain Management Model (Price *et al.*, 2007) the authors have produced a guide for wound pain assessment and management that has four levels: wound assessment, local wound management, wound pain assessment and wound pain management. The first two will be considered in Chapter 3 and their proposed wound pain assessment is summarised in Figure 2.2.

Good record keeping of the assessment is essential as a starting point to enable a treatment plan to be developed and to monitor its effectiveness.

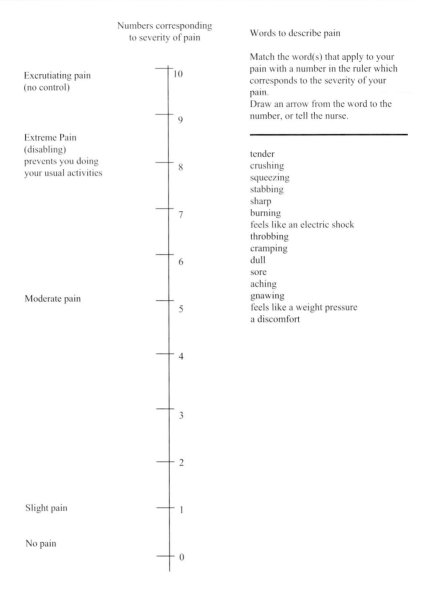

Figure 2.1   **A pain chart (from Bourbonnais, 1981, reproduced with permission)**

B: be aware of the cause
Most wounds cause pain to a greater or lesser extent and treatment of the underlying aetiology and promotion of healing will assist in alleviating pain. In addition, wound infection or skin problems associated with the wound will cause increased pain. Identifying such problems is essential both to promote healing and reduce pain. These issues are discussed in greater detail in later chapters of this book.

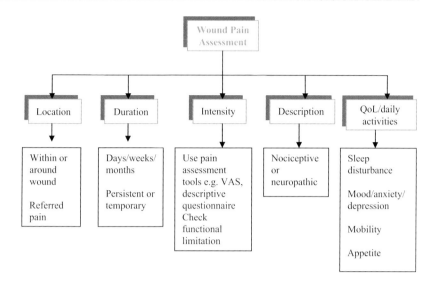

Figure 2.2 **Wound pain assessment (adapted from Wound Pain Management Model (Price *et al.*, 2007); reproduced with permission). QoL, quality of life; VAS, Visual analogue scale**

C: consider local treatment

Local treatment for pain may be more appropriate than systemic treatments as they reduce the risk of side-effects (Coutts *et al.*, 2008). A number of different strategies can be employed including the use of moist wound dressings, dressings that contain analgesia and topical analgesics. They will be discussed in detail in Chapter 4.

D: do we need systemic treatment?

Systemic treatment will be needed for large traumatic wounds, burn injury and surgical wounds. It will also be needed for patients with chronic wounds for whom local treatment has been found to be ineffective. Specific pain management protocols may be in place for some wound types. The World Health Organization pain relief ladder was originally developed for cancer pain, but is widely used for all types of pain. It uses three steps that move from non-opioids through weak opioids and on to strong opioids and uses adjuvant therapies such as muscle relaxants or steroids to enhance the effect of the analgesia (http://www.who.int/cancer/palliative/painladder/en/). Price *et al.* (2007) also suggest that tricyclic antidepressants or anticonvulsants may be more appropriate for neuropathic pain.

Effective pain management will only be achieved by careful initial assessment and ongoing re-evaluation of the effectiveness of the plan of care.

Sleeping

Most people consider sleep to be important as it provides a sense of refreshment and well-being. In recent years there has been considerable research on sleep and its effects. Sleep deprivation causes people to become increasingly irritable and irrational (Carter, 1985). They may complain of lassitude and loss of feelings of well-being. The sleep–activity cycle is part of the circadian rhythms. During wakefulness the body is in a state of catabolism. Hormones such as catecholamine and cortisol are released. They encourage tissue degradation to provide energy for activity, in particular, protein degradation occurs in muscle.

Growth hormone is secreted from the anterior pituitary during sleep and stimulates protein synthesis and the proliferation of a variety of cells including fibroblasts and endothelial cells (Lee & Stotts, 1990). Rose *et al.* (2001) reviewed the impact of burn injury on the sleep patterns of children and the need to aggressively treat growth hormone insufficiency. They speculate that improved sleep would improve growth hormone levels. However, Brandenberger *et al.* (2000) argue that the body is able to compensate during the day and the levels of growth hormone secreted over 24 hours remain much the same, regardless of any sleep deprivation.

There has been some reliance on animal studies to determine the impact of sleep deprivation and the surrogate measure, noise, on wound healing. Wysocki (1996) measured the impact of noise on wound healing and found that wounds healed more slowly compared with the controls. Two studies of wound healing seem to have contradictory results: Gümüstekin *et al.* (2004) found that sleep deprivation may delay wound healing; whereas Mostaghimi *et al.* (2005) found the reverse, that sleep deprivation appeared to make no difference to healing rates. It should be noted that these studies were undertaken on basically healthy animals and the findings may not be transferable to sick humans. Further studies, especially clinical studies, are needed to clarify the matter.

There is considerable evidence that sleep patterns are disturbed in hospital. A study exploring the experiences of older men in hospital found that patients were expected to fit in with the nurses work schedule rather than being able to follow their usual sleep routines (Lee *et al.*, 2007). Also, many patients are disturbed during the night, especially in the critical care unit. A review by Patel *et al.* (2008) noted that ventilated patients have been found to have up to 74 arousals and awakenings per hour. Friese *et al.* (2007) monitored the sleep patterns of 16 patients in a surgical critical care unit. They found that the patients had a mean of 8.2 hours sleep (standard deviation (s.d.) = 6.53) but that it was highly fragmented. Measurement of the stages of sleep showed that approximately 96% of sleep time was in superficial sleep and very little was actually the deep sleep of rapid eye movement (REM) sleep. Freedman *et al.* (1999) surveyed 203 patients immediately after discharge from different types of intensive care units and found that poor sleep quality was common to all intensive care units. They also found that sleep disruption was caused by human interventions, diagnostic testing and environmental noise. A further study from the same research centre investigated the impact of environmental noise on sleep. The sleep patterns of 22 medical patients in an intensive care unit were monitored for 24–48 hours continuously. Patients were found to sleep for short periods throughout a 24-hour time period with a mean number of sleep periods of 41 ± 28 and the mean length of a sleep nap was 15 ± 9 minutes. Overall, environmental noise was responsible for only 17% of sleep disturbances (Freedman *et al.*, 2001).

Other factors may also disturb sleep as shown in a survey by Southwell and Wistow (1995) of 454 patients and 129 nurses across a variety of wards in three hospitals. Half the patients had difficulty in sleeping through the nights and did not get as much sleep as they wished. Many of the patients complained that the ward was too hot and the mattresses were uncomfortable and they disliked having plastic covers on both mattresses and pillows. Pain and worry were also likely to make sleeping more difficult. A variety of factors were found to disturb sleep including: other patients making a noise, nurses attending other patients, telephones ringing, lights in the ward, nurses talking to each other or to patients, having treatment including medication, toilets flushing or commodes being used, nurses shoes making a noise. Christensen (2005) measured noise on a surgical ward and found that it did dip to reasonable levels at night time, but that 25% of the human noise came from the nurses' station. Nurses appeared to be unaware of the level of noise they made and the impact it had on the patients' psychological and physiological well-being.

Sleep-Enhancing interventions

Richardson *et al.* (2009) introduced a sleep promotion guideline on three wards in a teaching hospital. It included strategies such as turning telephone volume down or to vibrate at night and encouraging patients to use ear plugs or eye masks. After introduction of the guideline and a relevant education programme they found a significant reduction in peak noise levels although not in average noise levels.

Hospital routines can disrupt normal sleep patterns. The lights of a ward may go off late, around 23.00 hours and come on again at 06.00 hours (Southwell & Wistow, 1995). Patients are woken for their drugs and a drink. It seems not unreasonable for more flexibility be introduced with a reduction of the 06.00-hour drug round to a minimum and an arrangement not to wake those who would prefer to sleep later. Jarman *et al.* (2002) experimented with flexible morning and evening medication times and found that patients were able to sleep for longer. It should be possible, with careful planning, to provide an environment that is conducive to sleep and a patient who is comfortable and able to benefit from it.

Some people find their sleep disrupted because of pain. This may be acute pain following trauma or surgery or a more chronic pain relating to a long-standing illness or condition. Adequate pain control is essential. Pain is a resolvable problem (see also section on Pain). The position of patients may affect their comfort. It is helpful to ensure that the patient is in a comfortable position, with a bell close to hand.

During the night, many fears that are suppressed during the day come to the surface. Sleep may be disturbed because of a particular anxiety. Night-time is a quieter time on the ward. It may provide an opportunity for the nurse to sit and listen and allow patients to express their fears and anxieties. Once this has happened, the patient may be able to return to normal sleep patterns.

Hypothermia

Anaesthesia for major surgery can result in hypothermia as a result of decreased metabolic rate and impaired thermoregulation (Sellden, 2002). There is increased understanding of the impact even mild levels of intra-operative hypothermia can have on post-operative recovery.

Mahoney and Odom (1999) reviewed the outcome costs for mildly hypothermic patients compared with normothermic patients undergoing a range of operations. They were able to pool the findings of the studies and undertake a meta-analysis. They found that mildly hypothermic patients were more likely to require blood transfusions and to develop wound infections and the cost of these adverse outcomes ranged between $2500 and $7000. Flores-Maldonado et al. (2001) studied a prospective cohort of 290 surgical patients and found that mild peri-operative hypothermia was significantly associated with SSI. Similar results were found by Walz et al. (2006) in a study of 1446 patients following bowel surgery.

Qadan et al. (2009) studied the evidence relating to the impact of hypothermia on the wound and noted that hypothermia causes vasocon-striction in the skin in order to reduce heat loss, but also has the side-effect of causing wound hypoxia. In addition, hypothermia inhibits T-cell mediated antibody production and neutrophil activity thus reducing the ability to counter the bacterial challenge posed by the surgery. Using an in vitro model, the research team found that hypothermia significantly depressed monocyte activity, delayed clearance of TNFα and increased the release of IL-10. Again this has the result of reducing the ability to respond to bacterial invasion.

Plattner et al. (2000) tested an experimental warming bandage system and compared it with conventional gauze with elastic adhesive in 40 normothermic patients following elective abdominal surgery. The ex-perimental bandage consisted of an adhesive shell and a foam frame surrounding a clear window. A heated card was inserted into the frame approximately 1 cm above the wound surface and left in situ for 2 hours at a time. Oxygen tension was measured via a probe inserted 2–3 cm laterally to the incision. Their results were unexpected. They found that the oxygen tension was considerably lower in those receiving conventional dressings because of the pressure exerted by the elastic strapping. The warming device did not appear to benefit normothermic patients particularly, although it had potential for use for hypothermic patients.

Peri-operative hypothermia is associated with a higher incidence of wound infection. This is of particular relevance in surgery where there is already a high risk of infection such as abdominal surgery. It is less likely to be important in surgery with a low risk of infection, such as neurosurgery. There are also occasions when cooling the patient is appropriate during surgery such as during craniotomy.

Steroids

Glucocorticoids or corticosteroids are widely used in the treatment of inflammatory diseases. Although they produce effective anti-inflammatory outcomes, this can have a serious impact on wound healing. A review by Anstead (1998) has highlighted the fact that glucocorticoids affect every stage of the healing process. This includes overall effects such as the increased risk of infection and dehiscence in surgical wounds, although this is probably dose dependent. Grunbine *et al.* (1998) studied 73 patients who had had a steroid injection following surgery to the foot or ankle and compared the outcome with those who did not. The use of a single dose of steroids made no difference to healing rates.

Anstead (1998) summarised the effects of glucocorticoids on wound healing as follows.

- Inflammation is suppressed because of a reduction in the numbers of neutrophils and macrophages and an impaired ability to digest phago-cytosed material.
- Wound contracture is poor as a result of inhibition of fibroblast proliferation.
- There is reduced wound strength as collagen structure and cross-linking are affected.
- Epithelialisation is delayed and the cells are thin, producing a weak wound covering.

A study by Stojadinovic *et al.* (2007) explored the genomic effects of glucocorticoids on cultured human keratinocytes in an *in vitro* study. They found that glucocorticoids inhibited cell motility and also the expression of pro-angiogenic factor and vascular endothelial growth factor. They also found glucocorticoids suppressed production of transforming growth factor beta (TGFβ1 and 2) and MMP-1, -2, -9 and -10 and encouraged production of TIMP-2.

There has been some interest in the potential of vitamin A to counteract the unwanted side-effects of glucosteroids. Vitamin A has been found to restore a normal inflammatory response (Ehrlich *et al.*, 1972) and also epithelial regeneration, fibroblast proliferation and collagen content (Talas *et al.*, 2003). A more recent study suggests that androstenediol, an immune-regulating hormone, can reverse the effects of glucocorticoids in wound healing (Feeser *et al.*, 2009). However, both of these products have only been tested using animal models and clinical trials are needed to confirm the findings.

Radiotherapy

Radiation effectively destroys cancer cells as they are more radio-sensitive than normal cells. A dose high enough to kill cancer cells does not affect the surrounding cells. Using radiotherapy as an adjuvant treatment to surgery has been shown to have beneficial outcomes in tumour downstaging (Marks *et al.*, 2009). Radiotherapy is sometimes given before surgery to shrink the tumour and make it easier to remove and sometimes after surgery to eradicate all traces of cancer cells. However, an unwelcome side-effect is the impact on the healing surgical wound. For example, Bullard *et al.* (2005) found that there was a significantly higher incidence of wound complications for patients with rectal cancer who were treated with radiotherapy as well as undergoing surgery.

The timing of radiotherapy in relation to surgery seems to be a factor in the incidence of wound healing complications. Lin *et al.* (2001) found a history of radiotherapy was a factor in wound healing complications of breast reconstruction. Similar results were found by Wang *et al.* (2003) and O'Sullivan *et al.*, (2002), when comparing pre- and post-operative radiotherapy. Both studies found a significantly higher rate of wound healing complications when radiotherapy was given pre-operatively.

Akudugu *et al.* (2006) studied 46 cancer patients undergoing surgery. A total of 28 patients received pre-operative radiotherapy and the remaining 18 patients acted as the control group. Wound complications were found in 8 (29%) of the radiotherapy group compared with none in the control group. A larger study of a cohort of 216 head and neck cancer patients was undertaken by Halle at al (2009). They found those having pre-operative radiotherapy had a significantly higher incidence of total and partial flap failures compared with those who did not. They also found that there was a significant linear trend to increasing numbers of flap failures when there was a gap of more than 6 weeks between the last dose of radiotherapy and surgery. Marks *et al.* (2009) also found similar results in a group of 62 patients with rectal cancer. They found a wound complication rate of 25.6% (11 patients) in the radiotherapy group compared with 0% in the non-radiotherapy group.

The conclusions of these research groups were that the timing of radiotherapy must be based on the best course of action for treating the tumour. If it was appropriate, then post-operative radiotherapy was preferable. However, the wound healing problems are not considered an insuperable problem (Marks *et al.*, 2009) and Halle *et al.* (2009) suggest surgery should be timed to be within 6 weeks of the last radiotherapy treatment to allow optimum result.

Radiation may affect the healing of an existing wound or it may cause changes to the skin so that any later wound will heal slowly. The skin may show signs of damage from the radiation during treatment. This is known as a radiation reaction and will be discussed in Chapter 6.

Psychological care

Nurses have always excelled at the physical care of patients. It is only recently that the emotional needs of patients have been considered. Many situations may cause psychological distress. This may be described as stress. The physiological effects of stress and its effect on wound healing have already been described above. Factors causing psychological distress may be defined as stressors. Those that may be particularly associated with wounded patients will be discussed in this section. It should be noted that other factors, not addressed here, can also act as stressors.

Anxiety

Anxiety has been defined as 'a diffuse, unpleasant, vague sense of apprehension' (Sadock & Sadock, 2008). Anxiety is experienced by everyone at one time or another, especially when the future is uncertain, such as health problems or because of experiences such as admission to hospital. Much research has been undertaken into pre-operative anxiety and the following dimensions have been identified: fear of the unknown, fear of feeling ill and fear for life (Rosen *et al.*, 2008). Anxious patients have more severe pain and their blood pressure and cortisol levels have been shown to be higher (Augustin & Maier, 2003). Levandoski *et al.* (2008) monitored patients undergoing total abdominal hysterectomy that had been randomised to either diazepam 10 mg orally or placebo pre-operatively. They found a surgical site infection (SSI) rate of 25.8% (16/62) in the placebo group compared with 6.6% (4/61) in the diazepam group.

Assessment

Zigmond & Snaith (1983) have designed a simple questionnaire, known at the Hospital Anxiety and Depression Score (HAD) Score, that can identify the degree of stress being suffered and can be completed by patients. The questionnaire comprises a series of questions on topics such as whether an individual is worried or able to relax and enjoy watching television. There is a choice of four answers to each question such as 'most of the time' or 'seldom'. Most patients found it simple to use and were enthusiastic about the concept. Cole-King and Harding (2001) used the HAD score to identify stress in 53 patients with leg ulcers and found it to be useful research tool.

A more general assessment tool is the State Trait Anxiety Inventory (STAI-State) that has been used in a wide variety of situations (Spielberger, 1966). It is able to differentiate between the transient condition of 'state anxiety', where an individual finds a situation stressful and becomes anxious and the more general and long-standing quality of 'trait anxiety', where an individual has a predisposition to become anxious. The STAI-State has been widely used in studies to assess pre- and post-operative anxiety (for example: Ciccozzi *et al.*, 2007; Hermes *et al.*, 2007; Detroyer *et al.*, 2008; Bringman *et al.*, 2009; Badura-Brzoza *et al.*, 2009)

Nursing interventions

Much of the work addressing patient anxiety in relation to wounds has been undertaken in relation to elective surgery and the provision of effective pre-operative information. The UK Department of Health has produced a reference document that makes it clear that all patients have the right to understand their treatment and the risks involved (Department of Health, 2009). The role of the nurse is to ensure that each patient receives appropriate pre-operative information about the surgery and about what to expect in the post-operative period. Ideally, individual patients should be assessed for their level of anxiety so that relevant strategies can be determined. However, with many patients being admitted on the day of surgery, this may be difficult to achieve.

A number of studies have looked at the provision of written information prior to a surgical intervention and found it effective in reducing anxiety. Van Zuuren *et al.* (2006) suggest that the use of simple brochures could easily be implemented into practice. Eberhardt *et al.* (2006) suggest that it is the clarity of information that is important rather than the volume.

Multimedia approaches have also been used. Doering *et al.* (2000) assessed the impact of providing a videotape of a patient undergoing a hip replacement from time of admission to discharge, purely from a patient's perspective. One hundred patients were randomly allocated to either preparation group (shown the videotape) or a control group. They were assessed for levels of anxiety and pain for 4 days post surgery. The researchers found significantly lower levels of anxiety in the preparation group as well as a lower intake of analgesia, although there were no differences in the amount of pain. Similar results were found by Jlala *et al.* (2010) in a study of patients undergoing upper or lower limb surgery.

They developed a film of the patient's hospital journey and showed it to those randomised into the study group.

It is important to note that this type of information is not effective for all patients. A study of 463 patients undergoing cataract surgery found that use of a video and educational leaflet (study group) was not significantly different to use of an educational leaflet (control group). When asked for their preference of format 54% said they preferred verbal information, 47% the video and 36% printed. This may have been influenced by their age and poor vision (Tan *et al.*, 2005). In addition, provision of information can increase anxiety. Deyirmenjian *et al.* (2006) randomised patients about to undergo open heart surgery to either an educational session plus a tour of the cardiac surgery unit or standard care. They found only borderline statistical significance in favour of the intervention and suggested that cultural and social background may require a modification of educational strategies.

Alternative therapies

Some alternative therapies have been successfully used to assist patients in reducing anxiety. Music therapy has been used in the peri-operative period to reduce anxiety. A systematic review by Nilsson (2008) of 42 studies found that music had a positive effect in reducing anxiety in about 50% of cases. She found that the tempo of the music appeared to be important and that 60–80 beats per minute was the most effective. A later study by Bringman *et al.* (2009) compared music intervention with pre-operative midazolam 0.05–0.1 mg given orally and found the relaxing music to be significantly better in reducing anxiety.

Aromatherapy has been shown to reduce anxiety in a variety of settings (Braden *et al.*, 2009). A randomised study of 150 surgical patients compared standard treatment with Lavendin oils and sham aromatherapy. They found that the Lavandin group were significantly less anxious than the other groups. It must be noted that the sample size was small and larger studies are required to give a more definitive result.

Body image

Body image is the mental picture that a person has of him/herself. Body image is also closely associated with self-esteem. Ghaderi (2006) defined self esteem as 'the sense of contentment and acceptance that results from a person's appraisal of one's own worth, attractiveness, competence and ability to satisfy one's aspirations'. All patients with wounds have an altered body image that can have a profound effect on the person's self-esteem and motivation. Wounds that can have this effect are those resulting in disfigurement, such as burns, head and neck surgery, mastectomy, amputation and ostomies. Many patients will also be suffering from anxiety about their prognosis. Chronic wounds can also affect body image as shown in a study by Ebbeskog and Ekman (2001) who found that leg ulcer patients were embarrassed by their ulcer and bandages and hid it with clothing. The resultant stress can be so overwhelming that the patient may be unable to take in information, to share his feelings or to commence rehabilitation.

Nursing assessment

Neil (2001) has developed as assessment tool called the Stigma Scale to measure body image in relation to the skin. Users are asked to judge a series of 11 statements using a 5-point Likert scale. This is a promising approach, but a major limitation is that, as yet, the scale has been validated only by educated, mainly White, women and further work is required.

Nursing interventions

In the early stages, following the circumstances that led to an altered body image, some patients appear to be quite euphoric. This is because of simple relief at having survived. After a while the patient's attitude is likely to change. Common problems that can occur include:

- a sense of loss, similar to bereavement;
- anxiety related to diagnosis, especially if it is cancer;.
- loss of sexual function, which may be related to type of surgery or trauma or to either of the previous problems;
- withdrawal from social relationships with family or significant others, possibly due to a malodorous wound, or any of the previous problems.

The role of the nurse is to assist the patient to develop a re-integrated body image (Burgess, 1994). This may be achieved in a variety of ways. Perhaps the most important is accepting patients as they are, at whatever stage they have reached. Allowing patients to express their feelings and providing them with matter of fact information, such as an honest appraisal of the progress of the wound, is beneficial. Lazelle-Ali (2007) discussed how confusing it is for patients when healthcare professionals behave as though a wound is not malodorous when it is. It prevents patients discussing the problem openly and stops them feeling in control and able to participate in decision-making. It is also essential to include family and/or significant others in the patient's care and in any education programme. Good management of the wound should prevent odour or leakage, which helps to boost confidence.

In many areas, specialist nurses are employed to give help and support to patients, such as colorectal nurses or breast care nurses. They can build up a relationship with their patients that give the patient the confidence to express his feelings freely. In other circumstances, it may be a nurse who has a good relationship with a patient who is able to provide this service.

Other psychological problems

Fear

Fear is a common human experience that may be transitory or longer lasting. Illness may release many fears – fear of hospitalisation, fear of illness, fear of a life-threatening condition, fear of loss of affection of loved ones, fear of the mutilation of surgery. Such fear creates great stress within the sufferer. This may be made worse by the healthcare team failing to recognise when patients are experiencing fear and so not allowing them to express their feelings.

Grief

Grief is a normal process that allows adaptation to some major loss in a person's life. The wounded patient may have to come to terms with skin damage from burns, the loss of a limb or breast, or other types of mutilating surgery (see also Body Image, section). Kubler-Ross (1969) described various stages in the grief process that has led to broad acceptance of the concept of stages of grief. Although this is generally applied to bereaved persons it has relevance to those with the type of major wounds described above.

Maciejewski *et al.* (2007) explored the stage theory of grief in a longitudinal cohort study of 233 people following the death of a spouse or close family member from natural courses. They assessed the levels of disbelief, yearning, anger, depression and acceptance from 1 month to 24 months post loss. Acceptance was present throughout the study with the level increasing gradually to the end. Disbelief peaked at month 1 and then declined and the same pattern occurred for the other stages with yearning peaking at 4 months, anger at 5 months and depression at 6 months. Although it cannot automatically be assumed that all kinds of grief follow the same trajectory, this study still provides useful information for caring for grieving patients.

By listening to the patient and accepting without judgement, the nurse can assist in the grief process and thus reduce the amount of stress suffered. This may be particularly difficult during the stage of anger as the aggression expressed by the patient is often directed at the main caregivers. Understanding of the cause of the aggression will help the nurse deal with this stage of grief.

Powerlessness

Aujoulat *et al.* (2007) suggested people experience powerlessness when they are facing a situation with which they have not yet learned to cope and if they feel it is beyond their control. This is a feeling experienced by many hospital patients as they are placed in the subservient 'patient role'. A study of 33 nurses and 32 patients found that patients were concerned that unless they did as they were told their care would be compromised and they would be labelled as a difficult patient (Henderson, 2003). This study also found that nurses controlled the level of information given to patients as a form of control. A study of 42 former burn patients assessed their negative experiences while a patient and found that 67% experienced feelings of powerlessness (Wikehult *et al.*, 2008).

In a society where independence is prized, dependence on others may produce feelings of anger and frustration. Many patients remark that they feel a nuisance because they cannot care for themselves. It may also reduce the feelings of self-worth. A common attitude of elderly people when asked to participate in a research project is that they will do so – because it will help others. Such a contribution is important to them as they feel that, despite their physical limitations, they can still make a contribution to the good of society.

Nursing psychological assessment

Although the precise problem may vary, the assessment is the same.

- Observe body language – does the patient look relaxed, tense, fidgety, withdrawn, avoid eye contact, hypoactive, hyperactive?
- Conversation – does the patient talk excessively, not talk to anyone, ask questions, non-questioning?
- Do any of these terms describe the patient? Angry, confused, aggressive, confident, demanding, distrustful, anxious, fearful, critical, passive, depressed, euphoric, disorientated.

Katona and Katona (1997) proposed that a slightly different approach is required for assessing older people. They recommended the use of four simple questions.

- Are you basically satisfied with your life?
- Do you feel that your life is empty?
- Are you afraid that something bad is going to happen to you?
- Do you feel happy most of the time?

The patient would score a point for replying no to the first and last question and for replying yes to the middle two. Anyone with a score of two or more is probably depressed

Nursing interventions

Although nurse training is providing improved knowledge of psychological care, it may be more appropriate for the patient to have further help from others such as a clinical psychologist, a psychiatric trained nurse, a chaplain or a trained councillor.

Once the nurse has been able to recognise that the patient has some form of psychological problem, then strategies can be developed to allow the patient the opportunity of expressing his/her specific fears. Ensuring that they fully understand what is happening to them is especially important. Time may have to be allowed for 'casual' conversation, especially if the patient has few visitors. Assigning the same nurses to care for the patient can build up confidence. Involving the patient and, possibly, the family in all aspects of planning may be helpful. Patients with any sort of sensory loss will need orientation to the new surroundings.

Spiritual care

In recent years there has been increasing awareness of the importance of spiritual care within healthcare. Although much of it has centred around palliative care as is evidenced in the NICE guideline *Improving Supportive and Palliative Care for Adults with Cancer* (NICE, 2004), but it is seen to be wider than that as discussed in the paper *NHS Chaplaincy: Meeting the Religious and Spiritual Needs of Patients and Staff* (Department of Health, 2003). A survey by King *et al.* (1999) of 250 patients admitted to a London teaching hospital found that 79% of patients professed some form of spiritual belief, although not all engaged in a religious activity. A survey undertaken of 1.75 million patients in American hospitals found that emotional and spiritual care was seen as largely ineffective and as an area that was in considerable need of improvement (Clark *et al.*, 2003).

The National Institute for Health and Clinical Excellence (2004) suggests that healthcare professionals frequently fail to recognise when patients need spiritual support. Spirituality is a concept that many nurses find difficult to define and they may feel unsure of what is required. Spirituality should not just be put into the framework of religion. Everyone has spiritual needs whether they believe in a God or not. Spirituality can be defined as that within us that responds to the infinite realities of life. Four constructs of spirituality have been identified (Stranahan, 2008):

- meaning and purpose;
- inner strength for hoping and coping;
- transcendent relationships with God and others;
- religious practices.

If the spiritual needs of individuals are not met, or they experience a catastrophic event in their lives, the result is spiritual pain or distress, this acts as a stressor and thus can impact on wound healing. Kohler (1999) defined spiritual distress as the failure of giving meaning to one's life. In her study of French AIDS and cancer patients, Kohler found that nearly all of them expressed feelings of 'ill being' and raised questions about the meaning of life, death, pain or illness. Kawa *et al.* (2003) studied palliative care patients in Japan and described spiritual distress as consciousness of the gap between an individual's aspirations and their current situation. The patients in the study were distressed by the gap between their current situation and how they wanted to live, or how they wanted to die or how they wanted to maintain relationships with others. Buxton (2007) interviewed 22 patients in a UK teaching hospital with the aim of gaining greater clarity of the terms spiritual integrity and spiritual distress. He found that many of the patients defined their distress in terms of having lost a sense of their true identity. These feelings were echoed in a study of patients with lung cancer or heart failure who described a sense of displacement that made them question their value and place in the world (Murray *et al.*, 2007).

Cressey and Winbolt-Lewis (2000) worked with a group of chaplains and lay people to determine areas of potential distress where the patient can be left with feelings of isolation, fragmentation or despair. They are listed in Table 2.2. In the context of spiritual distress, acceptance also has significance. A patient may need reassurance that others, particularly family and friends, will accept him/her in the new role as a patient, especially if having to come to terms with a disfiguring wound. Finlay *et al.* (2000) suggests that

Table 2.2   **Potential causes of spiritual distress (based on Cressey and Winbolt-Lewis, 2000)**

Potential cause	Explanation
Being valued	Individuals need to feel loved and valued and have a sense of belonging. If this is not present, patients can feel isolated and fragmented
Finding meaning	Illness and suffering challenges preconceived ideas of the meaning of life and need to search for further meaning – until this is found the patient will suffer
Having hope	Hope is a major motivator and powerful life force. The loss of hope results in misery and melancholy
Emotions	Emotions are part of everyday life, but the distressed patient may express feelings of fear, doubt or despair
Having dignity	Loss of privacy and dignity can be very distressing as can a failure to respect aspects of the many different cultures in today's society
Truth and honesty	Everyone is entitled to truth and honesty but this needs to be expressed with compassion and insight. Denying patients this right may result in tensions within their family and a 'conspiracy of silence'
Good communication	Failures of communication can cause distress and even offence
Death, dying, bereavement and loss	This often links to the need to find meaning and patients may ask 'why me?'
Religion	Patients can be very distressed by the lack of opportunity to follow their usual religious observances
Culture	For some, cultural observances are intertwined with their religious beliefs, yet we often fail to recognise them

patients perceive that healthcare professionals are too busy to discuss concerns relating to spiritual matters and so only disclose their distress when it becomes severe.

Nursing assessment

Peterman *et al.* (2002) have developed a validated assessment tool to measure spiritual well-being, which it call the Functional Assessment of Chronic Illness Therapy-Spiritual Well-Being (FACIT-sp). The assessment tool measures a sense of meaning and peace and also the role of faith in illness. However, it has only been validated with cancer patients.

Steinhauser *et al.* (2006) suggest that a simple question of 'are you at peace?' can be used as a screening tool to determine if further assessment is required. They used it within an interview setting alongside the FACIT-sp tool on 248 patients with advanced serious illness. They found a significant correlation between peacefulness and the FACIT-sp subscales of purpose and faith.

Stranahan (2008) listed a number of objective signs indicative of spiritual distress that include:

- sleep disturbance;
- anger;
- crying;
- withdrawal;
- preoccupation;
- hostility;
- apathy.

The signs of spiritual despair include:

- loss of hope;
- refusal to communicate with loved ones;
- loss of spiritual belief;
- death wish;
- severe depression.

Nursing interventions

Cavendish *et al.* (2003) suggest that provision of spiritual care is part of nursing care, although nurses may not always be comfortable with the concept. Nurses are not always able to recognise the difference between spiritual needs and religious needs. Cressey and Winbolt-Lewis (2000) describe spiritual care as conveying to patients that they have value and are unconditionally regarded for who they are, regardless of illness, colour or creed.

The chaplaincy team are very much part of the multiprofessional team and can give valuable support to both the patients and staff by both listening, comforting and counselling when necessary. However, nurses need to have some understanding of the range of spiritual care activities. There can be no standardised nursing care as there is with post-operative physical care. In this situation, each patient must be cared for in the light of his/her unique needs. Fish and Shelly (1985) proposed the following activities: listening, empathy, vulnerability, humility and commitment.

- *Listening*: this is active listening, giving the patient full attention and noting all the non-verbal as well as verbal cues.
- *Empathy*: this allows the nurse to share the feelings of the patient without loosing objectivity. This is essential to enable the patient to consider alternatives.
- *Vulnerability*: as nurses enter into and share patients' feelings, they become vulnerable. This may be painful, but can also be rewarding.
- *Humility*: this is not easy, few people want to admit that they do not have the answers in their particular field. A sense of humility will enable nurses to see that they can learn from their patients. Humility also allows nurses to accept themselves and their patients in all their human frailty.
- *Commitment*: being with a patient through all the difficult times, sharing the pain as well as the joys, involves considerable commitment.

Several studies have investigated spiritual coping mechanisms. Dein and Stygall (1997) undertook a review of religion and chronic illness and found that religion was a positive coping mechanism. A qualitative study using grounded theory found that 13 Christian patients undergoing open heart surgery sought comfort through prayer. They used two strategies: praying themselves and enlisting others to pray for them, especially for the times when they were unable to pray (Hawley, 1998). Narayanasamy (2002) interviewed 15 chronically sick people (9 Christians, 2 Hindus and 4 no religious affiliation) and also found that prayer brought comfort as it gave both a sense of connectedness to God and also a sense of hope, strength and security. However, he only found this sense of connectedness to God (or Hindu deities) among the Christians and Hindus in his sample.

References

Akudugu JM, Bell RS, Catton C, Davis AM, Griffin AM, O'Sullivan B, Waldron JN, Ferguson PC, Wunder JS, Hill RP (2006) Wound healing morbidity in STS patients treated with preoperative radiotherapy in relation to in vitro skin fibroblast radiosensitivity, proliferative capacity and TGF-β activity. *Radiotherapy and Oncology*, **78**: 17–26.

Alberti K, Press C (1992) The biochemistry of the complications of diabetes mellitus. In Keen H, Jarrett J eds. *Complications of Diabetes*. London: Edward Arnold.

American Society of Anesthiologists (2002 ASA physical status classification system. Park Ridge, IL (http://www.asahq.org/clinical/physicalstatus. htm).

Andel H, Kamolz LP, Horauf K, Zimpfer (2003) Nutrition and anabolic agents in burned patients. *Burns*, **29**: 592–595.

Anstead GM (1998) Steroids, retinoids and wound healing. *Advances in Wound Care*, **11**: 277–282.

Augustin M, Maier K (2003) Psychosomatic aspects of chronic wounds. *Dermatology & Psychosomatics*, **4**: 5–13.

Aujoulat I, Luminet O, Deccache A (2007) The perspective of patients on their experience of powerlessness. *Qualitative Health Research*, **17**: 772–785.

Badura-Brzoza K, Zajac P, Brzoza Z, Kasperska-Zajac A, Matysiakiewicz J, Piegza M, Hese RT, Rogala B, Semenowicz J, Koczy B (2009) Psychological and psychiatric factors related to health-related quality of life after total hip replacement - preliminary report. *European Psychiatry: the Journal of the Association of European Psychiatrists*, **24**: 119–24.

Bartsch RH, Weiss G, Kastenbauer T, Patocka K, Deutinger M, Krapohl BD, Benditte-Klepetko HC (2007) Crucial aspects of smoking in wound healing after breast reduction surgery. *Journal of Plastic, Reconstructive & Aesthetic Surgery*, **60**: 1045–1049.

Bell L, Duffy A (2009) Pain assessment and management in surgical nursing: a literature review. *British Journal of Nursing*, **18**: 153–156.

Bjarnsholt T, Kirketerp-Møller K, Jensen PO, Madsen KG, Phipps R, Krogfelt K, Høiby N, Givskov M (2008) Why chronic wounds will not heal: a novel hypothesis. *Wound Repair & Regeneration*, **16**: 2–10.

Booi DI, Debats IB, Boeckx WD, van der Hulst RR (2007) Risk factors and blood flow in the free transverse rectus abdominis (TRAM) flap: smoking and high flap weight impair the free TRAM flap microcirculation. *Annals of Plastic Surgery*, **59**: 364–371.

Bourbonnais F (1981) Pain assessment: development of a tool for the nurse and patient. *Journal of Advanced Nursing*, **6**: 277–282.

Braden R, Reichow S, Halm MA (2009) The use of the essential oil Lavandin to reduce pre-operative anxiety in surgical patients. *Journal of Perianesthesia Nursing*, **24**: 348–355.

Brandenberger G, Gronfier C, Chapotot F, Simon C, Piquard F (2000) Effect of sleep deprivation on overall 24 h growth hormone secretion. *Lancet*, **356**: 1408.

Bringman H, Giesecke K, Thorne A, Bringman S (2009) Relaxing music as premedication before surgery: a randomised controlled trial. *Acta Anaesthesiologica Scandinavica*, **53**: 759–764.

Bucknall T, Manias E, Botti M (2007) Nurses' reassessment of pain after analgesic administration. *Clinical Journal of Pain*, **23**: 1–7.

Bullard KM, Trudel JL, Baxter NN, Rothenberger DA (2005) Primary perineal closure after preoperative radiotherapy and abdominoperineal resection has a high incidence of wound failure. *Diseases of the Colon & Rectum*, **48**: 438–443.

Burgess L (1994) Facing the reality of head and neck cancer. *Nursing Standard*, **8**: 30–34.

Burnett E (2009) Perceptions, attitudes and behaviour towards patient hand hygiene. *American Journal of Infection Control*, **37**: 638–642.

Buxton F (2007) Spiritual distress and integrity in palliative and non-palliative patients. *British Journal of Nursing*, **16**: 920–924.

Carter D (1985) In need of a good night's sleep *Nursing Times*, **81**: 24–26.

Cavendish R, Konecny L, Mitzeliotis C, Russo D, Luise B, Lanza M, Medefindt J, Bajo MA (2003) Spiritual care activities of nurses using Nursing Interventions Classification (NIC) labels. *International Journal of Nursing Terminologies and Classifications*, **14**: 113–124.

Cereceda FC, Gonzalez GI, Antolin JFM Garcia FP, Tarrazo ER, Suarez CB, Alvarez HA, Manso DR (2003) Detection of malnutrition on admission to hospital. *Nutricion Hospitalaria*, **18**: 95–100.

Chapman A. (1996) Current theory and practice: a study of pre-operative fasting. *Nursing Standard*, **10** (18) 33–36.

Chbinou N, Frenette J (2004) Insulin-dependent diabetes impairs the inflammatory response and delays angiogenesis following Achilles tendon injury. *American Journal of Physiology – Regulatory Integrative & Comparative Physiology*, **286**: R952 – 957.

Christensen M (2005) Noise levels in a general surgical ward: a descriptive study. *Journal of Clinical Nursing*, **14**: 156–164.

Ciccozzi A, Marinangeli F, Colangeli A, Antonacci S, Pilerci G, Di Stefano L, Varrassi G (2007) Anxiolysis and postoperative pain in patients undergoing spinal anesthesia for abdominal hysterectomy. *Minerva Anestesiologica*, **73**: 387–393.

Clark PA, Drain M, Malone MP (2003) Addressing patients' emotional and spiritual needs. *Joint Commission Journal on Quality & Safety*, **29**: 659–670.

Cole-King A, Harding KG (2001) Psychological factors and delayed healing in chronic wounds. *Psychosomatic Medicine*, **63**: 216–220.

Correia ML, Waitzberg DL (2003) The impact of malnutrition on morbidity, mortality, length of hospital stay and costs evaluated through a multivariate model analysis. *Clinical Nutrition*, **22**: 235–239.

Coutts P, Woo K, Bourque S (2008) Treating patients with painful wounds. *Nursing Standard*, **23**: 42–46.

Creedon SA (2006) Health care workers' hand decontamination practices. *Clinical Nursing Research*, **15**: 6–26.

Creedon SA, Slevin B, De Souza V, Mannix M, Quinn G, Boyle L, Doyle A, O'Brien B, O'Connell N, Ryan L (2008) Hand hygiene compliance: exploring variations in practice between hospitals. *Nursing Times*, **104**: 32–35.

Cressey RW, Winbolt-Lewis M (2000) The forgotten heart of care: a model of spiritual care in the National Health Service. *Accident & Emergency Nursing*, **8**: 170–177.

De Boer AS, Mintjes-de Groot AJ, Severijnen AJ, van den Berg JMJ, van Pelt W (1999) Risk assessment for surgical-site infections in orthopaedic patients. *Infection Control and Hospital Epidemiology*, **20**: 402–407.

Dein S, Stygall J (1997) Does being religious help or hinder coping with chronic illness? A critical review. *Palliative Medicine*, **11**: 291–299.

Demling RH (2005) The incidence and impact of pre-existing protein energy malnutrition on outcome in the elderly burn patient population. *Journal of Burn Care & Rehabilitation*, **26**: 94–100.

Demling RH (2009) Nutrition, anabolism, and the wound healing process: an overview. *Eplasty*, **9**: e9.

Department of Health (2003) *NHS Chaplaincy: Meeting the Religious and Spiritual Needs of Patients and Staff.* London: Department of Health.

Department of Health (2009) *Reference Guide to Consent for Examination or Treatment*, 2nd edn. London: Department of Health.

Detroyer E, Dobbels F, Verfaillie E, Meyfroidt G, Sergeant P, Milisen K (2008) Is preoperative anxiety and depression associated with onset of delirium after cardiac surgery in older patients? A prospective cohort study. *Journal of the American Geriatrics Society*, **56**: 2278–2284.

Deyirmenjian M, Karam N, Salameh P (2006) Pre-operative patient education for open-heart patients: a source of anxiety? *Patient Education and Counselling*, **62**: 111–117.

Dihle A, Bjølseth G, Helseth S (2006) The gap between saying and doing in postoperative pain management. *Journal of Clinical Nursing*, **15**: 469–479.

Doering S, Katzlberger F, Rumpold G, Hofstoetter B, Schatz DS, Behensky H, Krismer M, Luz G, Innerhofer P, Benzer H, Saria A, Schuesler G (2000) Videotape preparation of patients before hip replacement surgery reduces stress. *Psychosomatic Medicine*, **62**: 365–373.

Ebbeskog B, Ekman SL (2001) Elderly persons' experiences of living with a venous leg ulcer: living in a dialectal relationship between freedom and imprisonment. *Scandinavian Journal of Caring Sciences*, **15**: 235–243.

Eberhardt J, van Wersch A, van Shaik P, Cann P (2006) Information, social support and anxiety before gastrointestinal endoscopy. *British Journal of Health Psychology*, **11**: 551–559.

Ehrlich HP, Tarver H, Hunt TK (1972) Effects of Vitamin A and glucocorticoids upon inflammation and collagen synthesis. *Annals of Surgery*, **177**: 222–227.

Ejaz S, Insan-ud-din, Ashraf M, Nawaz M, Lim CW, Kim B (2009) Cigarette smoke condensate and total particulate matter severely disrupts physiological angiogenesis. *Food & Chemical Toxicology*, **47**: 601–614.

Elia M, Stratton R (2004) On the ESPEN guidelines for nutritional screening 2002. *Clinical Nutrition*, **23**:131–132.

Feeser VR, Menke NB, Ward KR, Loria RM, Diegelmann RF (2009) Androstenediol reverses steroid-inhibited wound healing. *Wound Repair & Regeneration*, **17**: 758–761.

Finlay IG, Ballard PH, Jones N, Searle C, Roberts S (2000) A person to have around. What value do patients want from a Hospice Chaplain? *The Journal of Health Care Chaplaincy*, **3**: 41–52.

Fish S, Shelley JA (1985) *Spiritual Care: The Nurse's Role.* Downers Grove, IL: InterVarsity Press.

Flores-Maldonado A, Medina-Escobedo C, Ríos-Rodríguez HMG, Fernández-Domínguez R (2001) Mild perioperative hypothermia and the risk of wound infection. *Archives of Medical Research*, **32**: 227–231.

Freedman NS, Gazendam J, Levan L, Pack AI, Schwab RJ (2001) Abnormal sleep/wake cycles and the effect of environmental noise on sleep disruption in the intensive care unit. *American Journal of Respiratory and Critical Care Medicine*, **163**: 451–457.

Freedman NS, Kotzer N, Schwab RJ (1999) Patient perception of sleep quality and etiology of sleep disruption in the intensive care unit. *American Journal of Respiratory and Critical Care Medicine*, **159**: 1155–1162.

Friese RS, Diaz-Arrastia R, McBride D, Frankel H, Gentilello LM (2007) Quantity and quality of sleep in the surgical intensive care unit: are our patients sleeping? *Journal of Trauma, Injury, Infection & Critical Care*, **63**: 1210–1214.

Gazzotti C, Arnaud-Battandier F, Parello M, Farine S, Seidel L, Albert A, Petermans J (2003) Prevention of malnutrition in older people during and after hospitalisation. *Age & Ageing*, **32**: 321–325.

Ghaderi A (2006) The foundation of the self and the assessment of self esteem. In: Columbus A ed. *Advances in Psychological Research* (vol. 44). New York: Nova Science Publishers, pp. 69–86.

Grunbine N, Dobrowolski C, Bernstein A (1998) Retrospective evaluation of post-operative steroid injections on wound healing. *Journal of Foot & Ankle Surgery*, **37**: 135–144.

Guigoz Y, Lauque S, Vellas BJ (2002) Identifying the elderly at risk for malnutrition. The Mini Nutritional Assessment. *Clinics of Geriatric Medicine*, **18**: 737–757.

Gümüstekin K, Seven B, Karabulut N, Aktas Ő, Gürsan N, Aslan S, Keles M, Varoglu E, Dane S (2004) Effects of sleep deprivation, nicotine and selenium on wound healing in rats. *International Journal of Neuroscience*, **114**: 1433–1442.

Günes UY (2008) A descriptive study of pressure ulcer pain. *Ostomy Wound Management*, **54**: 56–61.

Halle M, Bodin I, Tornvall P, Wickman M, Farnebo F, Arnander C (2009) Timing of radiotherapy in head and neck free flap construction – a study of post-operative complications. *Journal of Plastic, Reconstructive & Aesthetic Surgery*, **62**: 889–895.

Hamilton K, Spalding D, Steele C, Waldron S (2002) An audit of nutritional care delivered to elderly inpatients in community hospitals. *Journal of Human Nutrition and Dietetics*, **15**: 49–58.

Hamilton Smith A (1972) *Nil by Mouth*. London: RCN Publications.

Hannemann P, Lassen K, Hausel J, Nimmo S, Ljungqvist O, Nygren J, Soop M, Fearon K, Andersen J, Revhaug A, von Meyenfeldt MF, Dejong CH, Spies C (2006) Patterns in current anaesthesiological peri-operative practice for colonic resections: a survey in five northern-European countries. *Acta Anaesthesia Scandinavica*, **50**: 1152–1160.

Hawley G (1998) Facing uncertainty and possible death: the Christian patients' experience. *Journal of Clinical Nursing*, **7**: 467–478.

Haydock DA, Hill GL (1986) Impaired wound healing in surgical patients with varying degrees of malnutrition. *Journal of Enteral and Parenteral Nutrition*, **10**: 550–554.

Henderson S (2003) Poer imbalance between nurses and patients: a potential inhibitor of partnership in care. *Journal of Clinical Nursing*, **12**: 501–508.

Hermes D, Matthes M, Saka B (2007) Treatment anxiety in oral and maxillofacial surgery. Results of a German multi-centre trial. *Journal of Cranio-Maxillo-Facial Surgery*, **35**: 316–321.

Herruzo-Cabrera R, Lopez-Gimenez R, Diez-Sebastion J, Lopez-Acinero MJ, Banegas-Banegas JR (2004) Surgical site infection of 7301 traumatologic inpatients (divided in two sub-cohorts, study and validation): modifiable determinants and potential benefit. *European Journal of Epidemiology*, **19**: 163–169.

Howard P, Jonkers-Schuitema C, Furniss L, Kyle U, Muehlebach S, Ödlund-Olin A, Page M, Wheatley C (2006) Managing the patient journey through enteral nutritional care. *Clinical Nutrition*, **25**: 187–195.

Hunt A (1997) Assessment and planning for older people. *Nursing Times*, **93**: 74–78.

James GA, Swogger E, Wolcott R, Pulcini ED, Secor P, Sestrich J, Costeron JW, Stewart PS (2008) Biofilms in chronic wounds. *Wound Repair & Regeneration*, **16**: 37–44.

Jarman H, Jacobs E, Walter R, Witney C, Zielinski V (2002) Allowing the patients to sleep: flexible medication times in an acute hospital. *International Journal of Nursing Practice*, **8**: 75–80.

Jenner EA, Fletcher BC, Watson P, Jones FA, Miller L, Scott GM (2006) Discrepancy between self-reported and observed hand hygiene behaviour in healthcare professionals. *Journal of Hospital Infection*, **63**: 418–422.

Jlala HA, French JL, Foxall GL, Hardman JG, Bedforth NM (2010) Effect of pre-operative multimedia information on perioperative anxiety in patients undergoing procedures under regional anaesthesia. *British Journal of Anaesthesia*, **104**: 369–374.

Jones J, Barr W, Robinson J, Carlisle C (2006) Depression in patients with chronic venous ulceration. *British Journal of Nursing*, **15**: 17–23.

Katona CL, Katona PM (1997) Geriatric depression scale can be used in older people in primary care. *British Medical Journal*, **315**: 1236.

Kawa M, Kayama M, Maeyama E, Iba N, Murata H, Imamura Y, Koyama T, Mizuno M (2003) Distress of inpatients with terminal cancer in Japanese palliative care units: from the point of view of spirituality. *Supportive Care in Cancer*, **11**: 481–490.

Kaya E, Yetim I, Dervisoglu A, Sunbul M, Bek Y (2006) Risk factors for and effect of a one-year surveillance program on surgical site infection at a university hospital in Turkey. *Surgical Infections*, **7**: 519–526.

Kiecolt-Glaser JK, Loving TJ, Stowell JR, Malarkey WB, Lemeshow S, Dickinson SL, Glaser, R. (2005) Hostile marital interactions, pro-inflammatory cytokine production, and wound healing. *Archives of General Psychiatry*, **62**: 1377–1384.

Kiecolt-Glaser JK, McGuire L, Robles TF, Glaser R (2002) Emotions, morbidity and mortality: new perspectives from psychoneuroimmunology. *Annual Review of Psychology*, **53**: 83–107.

King L (2001) Impaired wound healing in patients with diabetes. *Nursing Standard*, **15**: 39–45.

King M, Speck P, Thomas A (1999) The effect of spiritual beliefs on outcome from illness. *Social Science & Medicine*, **48**: 1291–1299.

Koen FM, Hulst J, Hulst JM (2008) Prevalence of malnutrition in pediatric hospital patients. *Current Opinion in Pediatrics*, **20**: 590–596.

Kohler C (1999) The nursing diagnosis of spiritual distress, a necessary re-evaluation. *Recherche en Soins Infirmiers*, **56**: 12–72.

Kondrup J, Johansen N, Plum LM, Bak L, Højlun Larsen I, Martinsen A, Andersen JR, Baernthsen H, Bunch E, Lausen N (2002) Incidence of nutritional risk and causes of inadequate nutritional care in hospitals. *Clinical Nutrition*, **21**: 461–468.

Kubler-Ross E (1969) *On Death and Dying*, London: Macmillan.

Lan CC, Liu IH, Fang AH, Wen CH, Wu CS (2008) Hyperglycaemic conditions decrease cultured keratinocyte mobility: implications for impaired wound healing in patients with diabetes. *British Journal of Dermatology*, **159**: 1103–1115.

Lazelle-Ali C (2007) Psychological and physical care of malodorous fungating wounds. *British Journal of Nursing*, **16** (suppl): S16–S24.

Lee CY, Low LPL, Twinn S (2007) Older men's experience of sleep in the hospital. *Journal of Clinical Nursing*, **16**: 336–343.

Lee JO, Benjamin D, Herndon DN (2005) Nutritional support strategies for severely burned patients. *Nutrition in Clinical Practice*, **20**: 325–330.

Lee KA, Stotts NA (1990) Support of the growth hormone-somatomedin system to facilitate wound healing. *Heart Lung*, **19**: 157–163.

Legendre C, Debure C, Meaume S, Lok C, Golmard JL, Senet P (2008) Impact of protein deficiency on venous ulcer healing. *Journal of Vascular Surgery*, **48**: 688–693.

Levandoski R, Ferreira MBC, Hidalgo MPL, Konrath CA, da Silva DL, Caumo W (2008) Impact of preoperative anxiolytic on surgical site infection in patients undergoing abdominal hysterectomy. *American Journal of Infection Control*, **36**: 718–726.

Li D, Puntillo K, Miaskowski C (2008) A review of objective pain measures for use with critical care adult patients unable to self-report. *Journal of Pain*, **9**: 2–10.

Lin KY, Johns FR, Gibson J, Long M, Drake DB, Moore MM (2001) An outcome study of breast reconstruction: presurgical identification of risk factors for complications. *Annals of Surgical Oncology*, **8**: 596–591.

Loughlin DT, Arlett CM (2009) 3-Deoxyglucosone-collagen alters human dermal fibroblast migration and adhesion: implications for impaired wound healng in patients with diabetes. *Wound Repair & Regeneration*, **17**: 739–749.

Maciejewski PK, Zhang B, Block SD, Prigerson HG (2007) An empirical examination of the stage theory of grief. *Journal of the American Medical Association*, **297**: 716–722.

McGuire L, Heffner K, Glaser R, Needleman B, Malarkey W, Dickinson S, Lemeshow S, Cook C, Muscarella P, Melvin WS, Ellison EC, Kiecolt-Glaser JK

(2006) Pain and wound healing in surgical patients. *Annals of Behavioural Medicine*, **31**: 165–172.

Macpherson C, Aarons D (2009) Overcoming barriers to pain relief in the Caribbean. *Developing World Bioethics*, **9**: 99–104.

Mahoney CB, Odom J (1999) Maintaining intraoperative normothermia: a meta-analysis of outcomes with costs. *American Association of Nurse Anaesthetists Journal*, **67**: 307–308.

Manassa EH, Hertl CH, Olbrisch RR (2003) Wound healing problems in smokers and non-smokers after 132 abdominoplasties. *Plastic & Reconstructive Surgery*, **111**: 2082–2087.

Manias E, Botti M, Bucknall T (2006) Patients' decision-making strategies for managing post-operative pain. *Journal of Pain*, **7**: 428–437.

Marks JH, Valsdottir EB, DeNittis A, Yarandi SS, Newman DA, Nweze I, Mohiuddin M, Marks GJ (2009) Transanal endoscopic microsurgery for the treatment of rectal cancer: comparison of wound complication rates with and without neoadjuvant radiation therapy. *Surgical Endoscopy*, **23**: 1081–1087.

Mathus-Vliegen EM (2004) Old age, malnutrition and pressure sores: an ill-fated alliance. *Journals of Gerontology Series A-Biological Sciences & Medical Sciences*, **59**: 355–360.

Miller JT, Btaiche IF (2009) Oxandrolone treatment in adults with severe thermal injury. *Pharmacotherapy*, **29**(2): 213–226.

Mishriki SF, Law DJW, Jeffery PJ (1990) Factors affecting the incidence of postoperative wound infection. *Journal of Hospital Infection*, **16**: 223–230.

Moro ML, Carrieri MP, Tozzi AE, Lana S, Greco D (1996) Risk factors for surgical wound infections in clean surgery: a multicentre study. Italian PRINOS Study Group. *Annals of Italian Chirugia*, **67**: 13–19.

Mostaghimi L, Obermeyer WH, Ballamudi B, Martinez-Gonzalez D, Benca RM (2005) Effects of sleep deprivation on wound healing. *Journal of Sleep Research*, **14**: 213–219.

Mowe M, Bosaeus I, Højgaard Rasmussen H, Kondrup J, Unosson M, Rothenberg E, Irtun Ø (2008) Insufficient nutritional knowledge among health care workers? *Clinical Nutrition*, **27**: 196–202.

Murray SA, Kendall M, Grant E, Boyd K, Barclay S, Sheikh A (2007) Patterns of social, psychological and spiritual decline toward the end of life in lung cancer and heart failure. *Journal of Pain and Symptom Measurement*, **34**: 393–402.

Narayanasamy A (2002) Spiritual coping mechanisms in chronically ill patients. *British Journal of Nursing*, **11**: 1461–1470.

National Collaborating Centre for Women and Children's Health (2008) *Clinical Guideline: Surgical Site Infection*. London: RCOG Press.

National Institute for Health and Clinical Excellence (2004) *Improving Supportive and Palliative Care of Adults with Cancer*. London: NICE.

National Institute for Health and Clinical Excellence (2006) *Nutritional Support in Adults*. London: NICE.

National Pressure Ulcer Advisory Panel/European Pressure Ulcer Advisory Panel/(2009) *Clinical Practice Guidelines for the Prevention and Treatment of Pressure Ulcers*. Washington DC: NPUAP.

Nazarko L (2009) Potential pitfalls to adherence to hand washing in the community. *British Journal of Community Nursing*, **14**: 64–68.

Neil JA (2001) The Stigma Scale: measuring body image and the skin. *Plastic Surgical Nursing*, **21**: 79–81, 87.

Neumayer L, Hosokawa P, Itani K, El-Tamer M, Henderson WG, Khuri SF (2007) Multivariable predictors of post-operative surgical site infection after general and vacular surgery: results from patient safety in surgery study. *Journal of the American College of Surgery*, **204**: 1178–1187.

Nightingale F (1974) *Notes on Nursing, What it is and What it is Not*. Glasgow: Blackie & Son. (First published 1859).

Nilsson U (2008) The anxiety and pain reducing effects of music interventions: a systematic review. *AORN Journal*, **87**: 780–807.

Ochoa O, Torres FM, Shireman PK (2007) Chemokines and diabetic wound healing. *Vascular*, **15**: 350–355.

Olsen MA, Nepple JJ, Riew KD, Lenke LG, Bridwell KH, Mayfield J, Fraser VJ (2008) Risk factors for surgical site infection following orthopaedic spinal operations. *Journal of Joint & Bone Surgery – American Volume*, **90**: 62–69.

O'Sullivan B, Davis AM, Turcotte R, Bell R, Catton C, Chabot P, Wunder J, Kandel R, Goddard K, Sadura A, Pater J, Zee B (2002) Peroperative versus postoperative radiotherapy in soft-tissue sarcoma of the limbs: a randomised trial. *Lancet*, **359**: 2235–2241.

Pablo AM, Izaga MA, Alday LA (2003) Assessment of nutritional status on hospital admission: nutritional scores. *European Journal of Clinical Nutrition*, **57**: 824–831.

Parsons EP (1992) Cultural aspects of pain. *Surgical Nurse*, **5**: 14–16.

Patel KL (2008) Impact of tight glucose control on postoperative infection rates and wound healing in cardiac surgery patients. *Journal of Wound Ostomy Continence Nursing*, **35**: 397–404.

Patel M, Chipman J, Carlin BW, Shade D (2008) Sleep in the intensive care unit setting. *Critical Care Nursing Quarterly*, **31**: 309–318.

Patel MD, Martin FC (2008) Why don't elderly hospital inpatients eat adequately? *Journal of Nutrition, Health & Aging*, **12**: 227–231.

Perkins C (2004) Improving glycaemic control in a metabolically stressed patient in ICU. *British Journal of Nursing*, **13**: 652–657.

Peterman AH, Fitchett G, Brady MJ, Hernandez L, Cella D (2002) Measuring spiritual well-being in people with cancer: the functional assessment of chronic illness therapy-Spiritual Well-Being Scale (FACIT-sp). *Annals of Behavioral Medicine*, **24**: 49–58.

Pinsolle V, Grinfeder C, Mathoulin-Pelissier S, Faucher A (2006) Complications analysis of 266 immediate breast reconstructions. *Journal of Plastic, Reconstructive & Aesthetic Surgery*, **59**: 1017–1024.

Plattner O, Akca O, Herbst F, Arkilic CF, Fugger R, Barlan M, Kurz A, Hopf H, Werba A, Sessler DI (2000) The influence of 2 surgical bandage systems on wound tissue oxygen tension. *Archives of Surgery*, 135: 818–822.

Pracek JT, Patterson DR, Montgomery BK, Heimbach DM (1995) Pain, coping and adjustments in patients with burns: preliminary findings from a prospective study. *Journal of Pain and Symptom Management*, **10**: 446–455.

Pratt RJ, Pellowe C, Loveday HP, Robinson N, Smith GW, and the epic guideline development team (2001) The epic project: developing national evidence-based guidelines for prevention healthcare associated infections. Phase 1: guidelines for preventing hospital-acquired infections. *Journal of Hospital Infection*, **47** (supplement): S1–S82.

Pratt RJ, Pellowe CM, Wilson JA, Loveday HP, Harper PJ, Jones SRLJ, McDougall C, Wilcox MH (2007) Epic2: National evidence-based guidelines for preventing healthcare-associated infections in NHS hospital in England. *Journal of Hospital Infection*, **65** (supplement): S1–S64.

Prelack K, Dylewski M, Sheridan RL (2007) Practical guidelines for nutritional management of burn injury and recovery. *Burns*, **33**: 14–24.

Price P, Fogh K, Glynn C, Krasner DL, Osterbrink J, Sibbald RG (2007) Managing painful chronic wounds: the wound pain management model. *International Wound Journal*, **4** (suppl 1): 4–15.

Price PE, Fagervik-Morton H, Mudge EJ, Beele H, Ruiz JC, Nyström TH, Lindholm C, Maume S, Melby-Østergaard B, Peter Y, Romanelli M, Seppänen S, Serena TE, Sibbald G, Soriano JV, White W, Wollina W, Woo KY, Wyndham-White C, Harding KG (2008) Dressing-related pain in patients with chronic wounds: an international patient perspective. *International Wound Journal*, **5**: 159–171.

Pull ter Gunne AF. Cohen DB. (2009) Incidence, prevalence, and analysis of risk factors for surgical site infection following adult spinal surgery. *Spine*, **34**: 1422–1428.

Qadan M, Gardener SA, Vitale DS, Lominadze D, Joshua IG, Polk Jr HC (2009) Hypothermia and surgery: immunologic mechanisms for current practice. *Annals of Surgery*, **250**: 134–140.

Renwick P, Vowden K, Wilkinson D, Vowden P (1998) The pathophysiology and treatment of diabetic foot disease. *Journal of Wound Care*, **7**: 107–110.

Richardson A, Thompson A, Coghill E, Chambers I, Turnock C (2009) Development and implementation of a noise reduction intervention programme: a pre and post audit of three hospital wards. *Journal of Clinical Nursing*, **18**: 3316–3324.

Rico RM, Ripamonti R, Burns AL, Gamelli RL, DiPietro L (2002) The effect of sepsis on wound healing. *Journal of Surgical Research*, **102**: 193–197.

Rojas IG, Padgett DA, Sheridan JF, Marucha PT (2002) Stress-induced susceptibility to bacterial infection during cutaneous wound healing. *Brain, Behaviour & Immunity*, **16**: 74–84.

Rose M, Sanford A, Thomas C, Opp MR (2001) Factors altering the sleep of burned children. *Sleep*, **24**: 45–51.

Rosen S, Svensson M, Nilsson U (2008) Calm or not calm: the question of anxiety in the perianesthesia patient. *Journal of PeriAnesthesia Nursing*, **23**: 237–246.

Rosenberg CS (1990) Wound healing in the patient with diabetes mellitus. *Nursing Clinics of North America*, **25**: 247–261.

Royal College of Nursing (2005) *Perioperative Fasting in Adults and Children. An RCN Guideline for the Multidisciplinary Team*. London: RCN.

Royal College of Physicians, British Geriatric Society and British Pain Society (2007) *The Assessment of Pain in Older People: National Guidelines. Concise Guidance to Good Practice Series, No 8*. London: RCP.

Russell CA, Elia M (2008) *Nutrition Screening Survey in the UK in 2007*. Redditch: BAPEN (http://bapen.org.uk/pdfs/nsw/nsw.07_report.pdf).

Russo PL, Spelman DW (2002) A new surgical-site infection risk index using risk factors identified by multivariate analysis for patients undergoing coronary artery bypass graft surgery. *Infection Control & Hospital Epidemiology*, **23**: 372–376.

Sadock BJ, Sadock VA (2008) *Kaplan & Sadock's Concise Textbook of Clinical Psychiatry*, 3rd edn. Philadelphia: Lippincott, Williams & Wilkins, p. 236.

Schaeffer DF, Yoshida EM, Buczkowski AK, Chung SW, Steinbrecher UP, Erb SE, Scudamore CH (2009) Surgical morbidity in severely obese liver transplant recipients – a single Canadian centre experience. *Annals of Hepatology*, **8**: 38–40.

Sellden E (2002) Peri-operative amino acid administration and the metabolic response to surgery. *Proceedings of the Nutrition Society*, **61**: 337–343.

Soon K, Acton C (2006) Pain-induced stress: a barrier to wound healing. *Wound UK*, **2**: 92–101.

Sorensen J, Kondrup J, Prokopowicz J, Schiesser M, Krähenbühl L, Meier R, Liberda M (2008) EuroOOPS: and international, multicentre study to implement nutritional risk screening and evaluate clinical outcome. *Clinical Nutrition*, **27**: 340–349.

Sorensen LT (2003) Smoking and wound healing. *EWMA Journal*, **3**: 13–15.

Sorensen LT, Hemmingsen U, Kallehave F, Wille-Jorgensen P, Kjaergaard J, Moller LN, Jorgensen T (2005) Risk factors for tissue and wound complications in gastrointestinal surgery. *Annals of Surgery*, **241**: 654–658.

Sorensen LT, Karlsmark T, Gottrup F (2003) Abstinence from smoking reduces incisional wound infection: a randomised, controlled trial. *Annals of Surgery*, **238**: 1–5.

Sorensen LT, Zilmer R, Agren M, Ladelund S, Karlsmark T, Gottrup F (2009) Effect of smoking, abstension, and nicotine patch on epidermal healing and collagenase in skin transudate. *Wound Repair & Regeneration*, **17**: 347–353.

Sorensen LT, Toft B, Rygaard J, Ladelund S, Teisner B, Gottrup F (2010) Smoking attenuates wound inflammation and proliferation while smoking cessation restores inflammation but not proliferation. *Wound Repair & Regeneration*, **18**: 186–192.

Southwell MT, Wistow G (1995) Sleep in hospitals at night: are patients' needs being met? *Journal of Advanced Nursing*, **21**: 1101–1109.

Spielberger CD (1966). *Anxiety and Behavior*. New York: Academic Press.

Steingrimsson S, Gustafsson R, Gudbjartsson T, Mokhtari A, Ingemansson R, Sjogren J (2009) Sternocutaneous fistulas after cardiac surgery: incidence and late outcome during a ten-year follow-up. *Annals of Thoracic Surgery*, **88**: 1910–1915.

Steinhauser KE, Voils CI, Clipp EC, Bosworth HB, Christakis NA, Tulsky JA (2006) "Are you at peace?" One item to probe spiritual concerns at end of life. *Archives of Internal Medicine*, **166**: 101–105.

Stojadinovic O, Lee B, Vouthounis C, Vukelic S, Pastar I, Blumenberg M, Brem H, Tomic-Canic M (2007) Novel genomic effects of glucocorticoids in epidermal keraticocytes: inhibition of apoptosis, interferon-γ pathway and wound healing with promotion of terminal differentiation. *Journal of Biological Chemistry*, **282**: 4021–4034.

Stranahan S (2008) A spiritual screening tool for older adults. *Journal of Religion & Health*, **47**: 491–503.

Talas DU, Nayci A, Atis S, Comelekoglu U, Polat A, Bagdatoglu C, Renda N (2003) The effects of corticosteroids and vitamin A on the healing of tracheal anastomoses. *International Journal of Pediatric Otorhinolaryngology*, **67**: 109–116.

Tan JF, Tay LK, Ng LH (2005) Video compact discs for patient education: reducing anxiety prior to cataract surgery. *Insight*, **30**: 16–21.

Taylor SJ (1999) Early enhanced enteral nutrition in burned patients is associated with fewer infective complications and shorter hospital stay. *Journal of Human Nutrition & Dietetics*, **12**: 85–91.

Van Zuuren FJ, Grypdonck M, Crevits E, Vande Walle C, Defloor T (2006) The effect of an information brochure on patients undergoing gastrointestinal endoscopy: a randomised controlled study. *Patient Education and Counselling*, **64**: 173–182.

Vilar-Compte D. Rosales S. Hernandez-Mello N. Maafs E. Volkow P. (2009) Surveillance, control, and prevention of surgical site infections in breast cancer surgery: a 5-year experience. *American Journal of Infection Control*, **37**: 674–679.

Vuolo JC (2009) Wound-related pain: key sources and triggers. *British Journal of Nursing*, **18** (suppl): S20–S25.

Walz JM, Paterson CA, Seligowski JM, Heard SO (2006) Surgical site infection following bowel surgery: a retrospective analysis of 1446 patients. *Archives of Surgery*, **141**: 1014–1018.

Wang Z, Qiu W, Mendenhall WM (2003) Influence of radiation therapy on reconstructive flaps after radical resection of head and neck cancer. *International Journal of Oral & Maxillofacial Surgery*, **32**: 35–38.

Wasiak J, Cleland H, Jeffery R (2007) Early versus later enteral nutritional support in adults with burn injury. *Journal of Human Nutrition & Dietetics*, **20**: 75–83.

White R, Cutting K, Kingsley A (2006) Topical antimicrobials in the control of the wound bioburden. *Ostomy Wound Management*, **52**: 26–58.

Wikehult B, Hedlund M, Marsenic M, Nyman S, Willebrand M (2008) Evaluation of negative emotional care experiences in burn care. *Journal of Clinical Nursing*, **17**: 1923–1929.

Williams JZ, Barbul A (2003) Nutrition and wound healing. *Surgical Clinics of North America*, **83**: 571–596.

Wissing U, Ek AC, Unosson M (2001) A follow-up study of ulcer healing, nutrition and life situation in elderly patients with leg ulcers. *Journal of Nutrition, Health & Ageing*, **5**: 37–42.

Wolcott RD, Cox SB, Dowd SE (2010a) Healing and healing rates of chronic wounds in the age of molecular pathogen diagnostics. *Journal of Wound Care*, **19**: 272–281.

Wolcott RD, Rhoads DD, Bennett ME, Wolcott BM, Gogokhia L, Costerton JW, Dowd SE (2010b) Chronic wounds and the medical biofilm paradigm. *Journal of Wound Care*, **19**: 45–53.

Woo KY, Sibbald RG (2008) Chronic wound pain: a conceptual model. *Advances in Skin & Wound Care*, **21**: 175–188.

Woo KY, Sibbald G, Fogh K, Glynn C, Krasner D, Leaper D, Österbrink, Price P, Teot L (2008) Assessment and management of persistent (chronic) and total wound pain. *International Wound Journal*, **5**: 205–215.

Woodhouse A (2006) Pre-operative fasting for elective surgical patients. *Nursing Standard*, **20**: 41–48.

Wysocki AB (1996) The effect of intermittent noise exposure on wound healing. *Advances in Wound Care*, **9**: 35–39.

Zigmond AS, Snaith RP, (1983) The hospital anxiety and depression scale. *Acta Psychiatrica Scandinavica*, **67**: 361–370.

3 General Principles of Wound Management

Introduction

This chapter will discuss, in broad detail, the general principles of wound management. Specific care of chronic and acute wounds will be considered in later chapters. The products mentioned in this chapter will be described in more detail in Chapter 4.

The ability to make an accurate assessment of a wound is an important nursing skill. It should be carried out in conjunction with an assessment of the patient as discussed in Chapter 2. The aim of the assessment is two-fold. It will provide baseline information of the state of the wound so that progress can be monitored. It will also ensure that an appropriate selection of wound management products is made. Keast *et al.* (2004) consider that accurate and comprehensive wound assessment requires meticulous and consistent clinical observation. To that end, they have proposed a mnemonic 'MEASURE' to provide a framework for assessment (Keast *et al.*, 2004, Table 3.1). In addition, wound classification, the position of the wound and the environment of care also need to be determined. These factors provide the framework for wound assessment and will be discussed next, first wound classification, then the position of the wound, the environment of care followed by the MEASURE framework.

Wound assessment

Wound classification

Wounds can be classified as chronic, acute and post-operative wounds.

- *Chronic Wounds* can be defined as wounds that have failed to proceed through an orderly and timely reparative process to produce anatomic and functional integrity (Werdin *et al.*, 2009). Any wound could become chronic. However, typical examples are pressure ulcers and leg ulcers. Patients may have multifactorial problems that affect their ability to heal their wounds.

The Care of Wounds: A Guide for Nurses, Fourth Edition. Carol Dealey.
© 2012 Carol Dealey. Published 2012 by John Wiley & Sons, Ltd.

Table 3.1   **MEASURE: a framework for wound assessment (From Keast *et al.*, 2004)**

	Parameter	Parameter Content
M	Measure	Length, width, depth and area
E	Exudate	Quantity and quality
A	Appearance	Wound bed, tissue type and amount
S	Suffering	Pain type and level
U	Undermining	Presence or absence
R	Re-evaluate	Monitoring all parameters regularly
E	Edge	Condition of wound edge and surrounding skin

- *Acute Wounds* are usually traumatic injuries. They may be cuts, abrasions, lacerations, burns or other traumatic wounds. They usually respond rapidly to treatment and heal without complication.
- *Post-operative wounds* are intentional acute wounds. They may heal by first intention, where the skin edges are held in approximation. Sutures, clips or tape may be used. Some surgical wounds are left open to heal by second intention, usually to allow drainage of infected material. Donor sites are also open wounds.

There may be related factors to be considered when managing each of these types of wounds, such as the relief of pressure for pressure ulcers. The care of chronic wounds will be considered in Chapter 5 and of acute wounds in Chapter 6.

Traditionally, some wounds have been classified according to depth. This type of classification is widely used in the USA, but generally only used to describe burns or, occasionally, pressure ulcers in the UK. Wounds are described in relation to the tissues that are damaged or destroyed.

- *Erosion* is the term used to describe the loss of one or two layers of epithelial cells. There is no depth to this type of wound.
- *Superficial wounds* are wounds where the epidermis has been damaged.
- *Partial-thickness wound* is when the epithelium and part of the dermis is destroyed. Hair follicles and sweat glands are only partially damaged. This type of wound is sometimes subdivided into partial-thickness and deep partial-thickness wounds. When these wounds have a large surface area, hair follicles and sweat glands produce epithelial cells during the stage of epithelialisation that form islets of cells on the wound surface, thus speeding the healing process.
- *Full-thickness wounds* have all of the epidermis and dermis destroyed. Deeper tissues such as muscle or bone may also be involved. Healing may take longer to establish in these wounds.

The position of the wound

The position of a wound should be noted as part of the assessment. It may be an indicator of potential problems, such as risk of contamination in wounds in the sacral region, or problems of mobility caused by wounds on the foot. Another factor to consider is the fact that a dressing may stay in place very well on one part of the body but not on another.

The environment of care

Consideration must be given to the environment in which care is to be given as the management of a wound can be affected by the circumstances of the patient. For example, the timing of a dressing change may not be particularly important for a patient in hospital. However, for a patient at home, perhaps a young mother with children to get to school, timing may be critical. Flexibility may be important for a patient with a long-standing wound who has to return to work. It may be helpful to arrange for the occupational health nurse in his/her place of employment to carry out the dressing change, thus reducing the frequency of clinic attendance. Not all wound management products are available in the community. Hospital nurses need to ensure that the product selected can be continued after discharge home. If a non-skilled person is to provide some of the wound care for a patient, adequate time must be allowed for teaching the individual appropriate routines. Adequate monitoring of care must also be established.

M = Measure

The size and shape of a wound may alter during the healing process. In the early stages as necrotic tissue and/or slough are removed, the wound appears to increase in size because the actual extent of the wound was originally masked by the necrotic tissue. Monitoring of wound shape is important to aid in dressing selection. A cavity wound requires a different dressing to a shallow wound. Some dressings are not appropriate for use if there is a sinus present. Accurate nursing records are essential for monitoring progress.

This section considers the various ways that a measurement of a wound may be undertaken. Some of them are not really appropriate for use in busy areas, but may have a value in a research study. Others are very expensive and so not available for most nurses. Whatever measurement is used, it should be done on a regular basis, the frequency depending on the type of wound. Chronic wounds should be measured every 2–4 weeks. Little change is likely to be seen by more frequent measurement, whereas acute wounds progress much more rapidly. Measurement should be done at each dressing change.

Simple linear measurement

The very simplest method of measuring a wound is to measure it at its greatest length and breadth and to measure the depth if appropriate. A small study by Langemo *et al.* (2008) compared four different methods for measuring a wound using a ruler and then calculated the wound surface area by multiplying the two lengths together. The researchers found that the most accurate method was the following: with a head-to-toe orientation, the longest length head-to-toe, and the widest width side-to-side, perpendicular (90-degree angle) to length. It is important that these measurements are taken on the perpendicular as Langemo *et al.* (2008) found that if they were just taken on the head-to-toe/side-to-side orientation there was over 70% overestimation of wound size with some wound shapes. They also recommend that everyone uses the same method for measuring a wound to ensure more accurate comparisons. If a wound is a relatively regular shape, then this can be a fairly successful method. It is also likely to be more accurate if the wound edges are marked to indicate the measurement points. A probe can be used if the wound is a very irregular shape or has sinus formation.

There are several drawbacks to using this type of measurement. Goldman and Salcido (2002) suggest that the method has limited sensitivity to changes in wound size and it also provides limited information about the shape of a wound. The accuracy of measurements may be rather doubtful if it is done by a great many people. The more people involved, the greater the risk of the measurement not being on the same spot each time. It is fair to state that even if the same person does the measurement each time, it still may not be replicated accurately. This is known as sampling error. If necrotic tissue or slough is present, the true wound size will become apparent as debridement occurs. Wound measurement will show that the wound has increased in size and can give a misleading picture of wound progress. Measurement gives no indication of wound appearance.

Overall comment: linear measurement is easy to undertake and cheap. There are limitations with its accuracy, but accuracy can be improved if the same method of measurement is used each time. More comprehensive data would be obtained if used in conjunction with a nursing chart.

Measurement of surface area

Flanagan (2003) reviewed the varying methods of wound measurement and found that measuring true surface area and monitoring the percentage reduction of wound surface area over time are the most useful methods. The most frequently used system for surface area measurement is that of tracing a wound. A variety of materials may be used, the commonest being acetate paper. One presentation of acetate paper is the lesion measure, samples of which are supplied by several dressing manufacturers. They are usually fairly small sheets with a series of circles on them. The centre circle is 1 cm in diameter and is surrounded by concentric circles that increase in size by 2-cm increments. This gives some estimate of measurement in the tracing.

Flanagan (2003) noted that errors can occur when undertaking wound tracings, particularly in identifying the wound margin. She suggested that establishing a simple protocol could help to improve accuracy. As with wound measurement, the tracing will show the increase or decrease in size without any explanation, as it does not provide information on wound appearance or depth.

The surface area of a wound can be calculated quite accurately by placing the tracing over squared paper and counting the number of whole squares. Squares that are at least 50% within the tracing are included in the total, but those of less than half are discounted (Gethin & Cowan, 2006). Successive tracings can be compared to show any difference in wound size. If necrotic tissue or slough is present then an initial increase in size will occur as debridement progresses.

More sophisticated computerised methods are also available, but less widely used. Keast et al. (2004) described a portable digital tablet (PDT, Visitrak™) that can be used in conjunction with wound tracings. A tracing can be placed on the digital tablet and a special stylus used to trace over the wound outline. The system calculates the surface area and percentage reduction in wound size from previous measurements.

Another system is digital image analysis (DIA), which uses a digital photograph and computerised image processing system. A photograph is taken and downloaded onto a computer where the programme calculates the wound surface area. It must, however, be noted that there is potential for inaccuracy when using a system involving a digital camera if the wound is over a curved part of the body such as the leg. One of the earliest examples is the Verge Videometer™ (VeV), but other versions are also available.

Several studies have been undertaken to compare the different methods of measuring wound surface area. In a small retrospective study Gethin and Cowan (2006) compared wound tracings with PDT and found no significant difference in measurements of wounds that were less than 10 cm^2. However, there was a significant difference in the two forms of measurement in larger wounds. Haghpanah et al. (2006) compared linear, PDT and DIA for accuracy and reliability of measurement of wound surface area. They found that the linear method was the least accurate and that DIA was slightly better than PDT for the measurement of large wounds and that PDT performed slightly better than DIA when measuring small wounds.

Shaw et al. (2007) compared PDT, DIA and elliptical measurement in 16 patients with diabetic foot ulcers. Elliptical measurements were obtained by using linear measurements and calculating the surface area using the formula πab. They found that PDT quick and easy to use, but unable to measure wounds smaller than 25 mm^2 accurately. The elliptical method was also quick and easy to use, but it was found to significantly underestimate wound size in smaller wounds. The DIA method was found to be repeatable, but the researchers were uncertain as to its validity.

Sugama *et al.* (2007) undertook a small study of the efficiency and convenience of the PDT using assessments of pressure ulcers. They tested intra- and inter-rater reliability and found it to be excellent (reliability coefficient = 0.99). They tested validity by comparing the measurements of 30 pressure ulcers with DIA and found a significantly strong positive correlation between the two. However, it was significantly faster to obtain a wound measurement using PDT compared with DIA.

A more recent development is the use of a colour-based image analysis algorithm to analyse surface area from photographs taken with a simple digital camera. Papazoglou *et al.* (2010) used photographs taken of 15 diabetic foot ulcers to test their algorithm. They found it to be a valid form of measurement except for wounds less than 1 cm^2.

Overall comment: measuring wound surface area allows wound progress to be monitored. There are limitations in all the methods currently available. In everyday practice, nurses are unlikely to have access to digitised equipment and so will be using simple methods like wound tracing. As long as the methods are standardised, regular tracings will provide reasonable information on the progress of a wound.

Measuring volume

When wounds are deep, it may be useful to measure wound volume. de la Brassinne *et al.* (2006) found measuring wound volume as well as surface area in a study of leg ulcers enhanced their knowledge of the progress of the wounds in the study. They found that reduction in wound volume could be detected at day 7 whereas reductions in wound surface area were only clearly apparent at day 28 in their study.

Theoretically, it is possible to calculate the volume by measuring the wound depth (using a sterile swab) and multiplying by the surface area. However, there are inherent errors in this method (Goldman & Salcido, 2002). Deep wounds are rarely cuboid in shape, may not have a uniform depth and sinus formation or undermining may be present. If the base of the wound is filled with necrotic debris, it must first be cleansed from the wound before undertaking any measurements (Keast *et al.*, 2004).

de la Brassinne *et al.* (2006) used an alginate dental mould to create a mould of leg ulcers in their study. They then weighed the mould to determine wound volume. This is straightforward in relatively shallow ulcers, but may be more difficult in deep wounds with undermining and totally unsuitable in very large wounds. Barber (2008) has described a computerised tool that uses a simple formula to calculate wound volume. However, although she has used it in clinical practice its validity and reliability has not been tested.

Overall comment: the most practical method of monitoring changes in wound volume is to measure and record the depth at the deepest part of the wound and to note the amount of dressing required to fill the cavity.

E = Exudate

The amount of wound exudate varies during the healing process. In a normally healing wound, there is considerable exudate at the inflammatory stage and very little at epithelialisation. A copious exudate may indicate a prolonged inflammatory stage or infection. A World Union of Wound Healing Societies (WUWHS) consensus document discusses the role of wound exudate and suggests that exudate promotes healing in the healing wound but seems to have the opposite effect on wounds with delayed healing (WUWHS, 2007). Further research is required to determine to role of wound exudate in delayed healing.

Assessment of the levels of wound exudate is important as it is an indicator for wound progress or complication as well as affecting dressing selection. For example, high levels of exudate production may indicate wound inflammation or infection (WUWHS, 2007). Falanga (2000) proposed a scoring system for wound exudate quantity that provides some qualification with the aim of achieving standardisation. Thus

1 = minimal (dressings last up to 1 week)
2 = moderate (dressings changed every 2–3 days)
3 = heavy (dressings changed at least daily)

An alternative method to quantify exudate was used by Browne *et al.* (2004a) in a multicentre study assessing dressing performance in the presence of heavy exudate (called the WRAP study). The research team used the TELER® system of clinical indicators (Le Roux, 1993) to measure exudate leakage. A clinical indicator is an ordinal measuring scale with six reference points that measure change. Each reference point is clinically significant with zero being the worst possible outcome and five the best. Table 3.2 shows the clinical indicator for exudate leakage when the planned frequency of dressing change is every 2 days. Exudate is considered to leak if it strikes through the outer bandage or strapping. Although this system measures exudate leakage rather than exudate amount, it still has clear clinical relevance.

A relatively new concept for measuring exudates levels is a disposable sensor that can be left in place on the wound under the dressing (McColl *et al.*, 2009). The electrodes within the sensor have tags that are left outside of the dressing or bandage and taped down. When the moisture level is to be read the tags are freed and attached to a portable meter. Readings range across five moisture bands from dry to wet. In a small study of 15 patients with venous leg ulcers, the meter readings were compared with clinical

Table 3.2 **Exudate leakage using TELER indicator (from Browne *et al.* (2004a), reproduced by kind permission of Longhand Data Ltd)**

Code	Exudate leakage
5	No leakage between routine/planned dressing change
4	Exudate leakage within 2 hours of next dressing change
3	Exudate leakage within 8 hours of next dressing change
2	Exudate leakage within 24 hours of dressing change
1	Exudate leakage within 8 hours of dressing change
0	Exudate leakage within 2 hours of dressing change

judgement and found to be comparable (McColl *et al.*, 2009). Further study is required to determine the overall value of this type of monitor.

There is benefit in using clearly defined terminology to describe exudate quality/colour. It may be of particular importance in post-surgical wounds where is potential risk of post-operative bleeding. Therefore the terms serous, serosanguinous, sanguinous, seropurulent and purulent may be useful.

Odour is much more difficult to measure in any objective way. Odour may be indicative of infection, but wound odour also increases as necrotic tissue debrides by autolysis. Some dressings such as hydrocolloids may produce a foul smelling odour when they are removed. It must also be remembered that many patients are distressed by wound odour and may feel embarrassment, disgust or shame (Hack, 2003). In a further paper on the WRAP project, Browne *et al.* (2004b) describe a clinical indicator to quantify odour (Table 3.3). It provides a simple and easily used measure that resonates with clinical experience. Browne *et al.* (2004b) used it in conjunction with a patient focused indicator to determine the impact of odour on the patient, thus making it an even more powerful tool.

Table 3.3 **TELER indicator to quantify odour (from Browne *et al.* (2004b), reproduced by kind permission of Longhand Data Ltd)**

Code	Odour
5	No odour
4	Odour is detected on removal of the dressing
3	Odour is evident on exposure of the dressing
2	Odour is evident at arms length from the patient
1	Odour is evident on entering room
0	Odour is evident on entering house/ward/clinic

A = Appearance

The appearance of the wound gives an indication of the stage of healing that it has reached or of any complication that may be present. Open wounds or wounds healing by second intention can be categorised as:

- necrotic;
- infected;
- sloughy;
- granulating;
- epithelialising;

Some wounds may be seen to have more than one category and so present as 'mixed' wounds. Before assessing a wound, the nurse should ensure that all the old dressing has been removed. Many modern dressings form a gel, which may give a misleading impression of the wound unless it is first cleansed away.

Necrotic wounds (Figure 3.1)

When an area of tissue becomes ischaemic for any length of time, it will die. The area may form a necrotic eschar or scab. This can be black or brown in colour. Some necrotic tissue may present as a thick slough that can be brown, grey or off-white. When assessing these wounds it is important to remember that the wound may be more extensive than is apparent. The eschar or slough masks the true size of the wound. Intervention is needed for these wounds to heal.

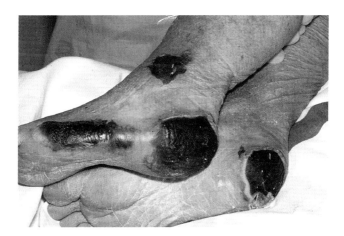

Figure 3.1 **Necrotic wounds**

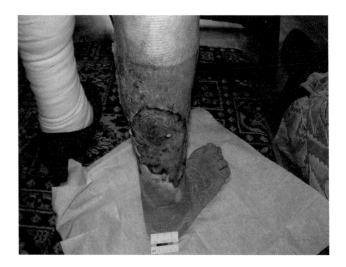

Figure 3.2 **An infected wound**

Infected wounds (Figure 3.2)

All wounds are colonised with bacteria. This does not delay healing or mean that wounds will automatically become infected. If infection occurs, there should be clinical signs of infection present. The classical signs of infection are pain, heat, swelling, erythema and pus. The signs may vary slightly according to the bacteria causing the infection. Usually there is localised erythema or redness, it may be restricted to just one part of the wound, such as at one end of a suture line, or it may spread to a large area around the wound. Associated with the erythema is heat in the adjacent tissue that will also feel hotter than the skin at a distance from the wound. Oedema or swelling around the wound is also present. The colour of the exudate and the slough on the wound surface depends on the bacteria causing the infection. There is usually a heavy exudate as the body rushes extra neutrophils and macrophages to the affected area and also tries to 'wash' the bacteria away. The exudate may have an offensive odour and can be the first indication of infection. Patients may also complain of increased pain.

However, chronic wounds do not always have such clear clinical signs. Cutting and Harding (1994) proposed additional criteria to those discussed above:

- delayed healing (compared with expected rate, may be for other reasons);
- discolouration: relates to wound bed;
- friable granulation tissue that bleeds easily;
- unexpected pain or tenderness;
- pocketing or bridging at the base of the wound;

- abnormal odour;
- wound breakdown.

A Delphi study, using an international, multiprofessional group of experts, was undertaken to generate criteria for infection in six wound types (European Wound Management Association, 2005). The findings showed that some criteria were deemed to be common to all wound types: cellulites, malodour, pain, delayed healing or deterioration of the wound. The other criteria listed above were seen as less important and pocketing or bridging was not mentioned at all.

A consensus document on the principles of best practice in relation to wound infection provides useful guidance on the triggers for suspecting wound infection for both acute and chronic wounds (Medical Education Partnership Ltd, 2008). It includes all the features listed above and adds the additional signs that can be found in spreading infection and then systemic infection.

The concept of critical colonisation is one that has been discussed by a number of authors, for example Sibbald *et al.* (2006) and White (2006). It was initially described by Davis (1996) as a 'multiplication of organisms without invasion but interfering with wound healing'. In other words, wound healing is delayed but there are no overt signs of infection. However, some authors (Jørgensen *et al.*, 2006; Sibbald *et al.*, 2006) have cited the clinical signs of critical colonisation to include:

- delayed healing;
- increased serous or purulent exudate;
- malodour;
- increased wound pain;
- dusky red granulation tissue.

All of these clinical signs have also been used to describe infection. Clearly, there is need for further investigation and debate in this area.

Traditionally we have thought of bacteria as planktonic or free-floating and this is the case for some bacteria, but there is increasing interest in the role of biofilms in wound infection. Biofilms have been defined as a colony of bacteria that has adhered to the wound surface and is encased within an extracellular polymeric matrix (EPS), which is produced by the bacteria (Hill *et al.*, 2010). The biofilm may comprise a single bacteria or a wide range of bacteria and once established may be difficult to remove. They are more commonly found in chronic wounds than acute wounds as shown in a study by James *et al.* (2008) who found that 30 of 50 chronic wounds (60%) compared with 1 of 16 acute wounds (6%) contained a biofilm. Bjarnsholt *et al.* (2008) put forward the hypothesis that chronic wounds are kept in a state of prolonged inflammation because the biofilm develops and excretes virulence factors that prevent neutrophils penetrating and destroying

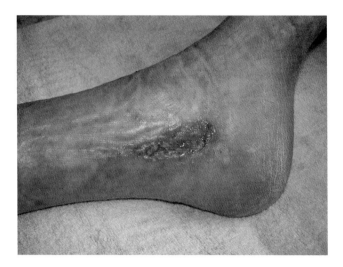

Figure 3.3   **A sloughy wound**

the bacteria. They suggest that the biofilm could produce substances capable of eliminating neutrophils which would account for the high levels of matrix metalloproteinases (MMPs) in chronic wounds. At present identification of biofilms has mostly been by taking tissue samples for electron scanning microscopy. It is not possible to identify them visually when assessing a wound.

Sloughy wounds (Figure 3.3)
Slough is typically a white/yellow colour. It is most often found as patches on the wound surface, although it may cover large areas of the wound. It is made up of dead cells that have accumulated in the exudate. It can be related to the end of the inflammatory stage in the healing process. Neutrophils have only a short lifespan and may die faster than they can be removed. Given the right environment for healing, the macrophages are usually capable of removing the slough and it disappears as healing progresses. Harding (1990) refers to a yellow fibrinous membrane that develops on the surface of some wounds. It is not stuck fast but can be easily removed. The membrane has no effect on healing and recurs if removed. He describes it as a variant on the normal.

Granulating wounds (Figure 3.4)
Granulation tissue was first described by John Hunter in 1786. It relates quite well to the stage of reconstruction in the healing process. The wound colour is red. The tops of the capillary loops cause the surface to look granular, hence the name. It should be remembered that the walls of the capillary loops are very thin and easily damaged, which explains why these

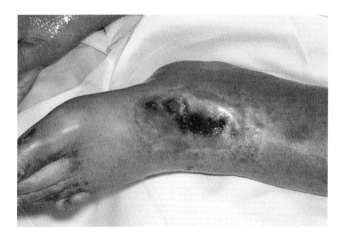

Figure 3.4   **A granulating wound**

wounds bleed easily. Regular, careful measurement will show a reduction in wound volume as the cavity fills with new tissue and contracts inwards.

Epithelialising (Figure 3.5)

As the epithelia at the wound margins start to divide rapidly, the margin becomes slightly raised and has a bluey-pink colour. As the epithelia spread across the wound surface, the margin flattens. The new epithelial tissue is a pinky-white colour. In shallow wounds with a large surface area, islets of epithelialisation may be seen. The progress of epithelialisation may be easily identified as the new cells are a different colour from those of the surrounding tissue.

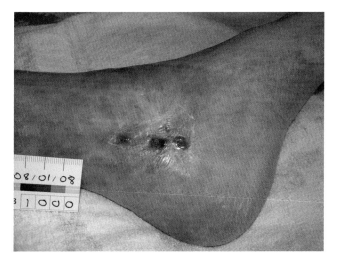

Figure 3.5   **An epithelialising wound**

Recording wound appearance

Wound appearance can be recorded in a number of ways. The simplest is the written word, however, this is also likely to be the most subjective and open to misuse and misinterpretation. Common examples are 'wound healing well' or 'wound a bit sloughy'. Neither of these assessments have a great deal of value when trying to accurately monitor wound progress. In an attempt to overcome this problem, some investigators use percentages to determine the quantity of each tissue type on the wound surface. However, it should be used with some caution as not all nurses and doctors can necessarily identify all the tissue types. A very small study of 16 doctors and nurses by Stremitzer *et al.* (2007) found that over 50% were unable to identify necrotic or granulation tissue in a diabetic foot ulcer. It would seem that an education programme is likely to be required before introducing this type of assessment into a clinical area.

The old adage 'a picture is worth a thousand words' may not be strictly true in relation to photographs of wounds, but photography does address some of the criticisms of the previous methods. A photograph provides clear evidence of the appearance of a wound and some suggestion of its size, especially if a rule is incorporated to provide a scale. Houghton *et al.* (2000) investigated validity and reliability of using photographs to assess wound status in comparison to a pressure ulcer assessment tool. They concluded that it was a valid and reliable tool for assessing wounds on the trunk and lower extremities. Regular photographs can provide real encouragement to both patients with chronic wounds and their carers. It should be remembered that the depth of a wound is not demonstrated in a photograph, as it does not accurately record wounds on curved surfaces.

Increasingly digital cameras are being used in clinical practice. They are gradually improving in quality and becoming cheaper. Many have impressive technical features, but they are not able to produce reproducible images with regards to the colours within the image (Van Pouche *et al.*, 2010). These differences may be further increased if the lighting or camera setting also differs when taking further images. In order to correct this problem, Van Pouche *et al.* (2010) have proposed an automatic colour calibration algorithm that can be used with commercially available digital cameras.

Not all nurses have access to a camera. It may be possible to obtain one on a short-term loan if a dressing trial is being undertaken. Several factors need to be considered if the purchase of a camera is planned.

- How can pictures be taken from the same angle and distance each time?
- How will patient consent be recorded? Some hospitals have a consent form for photography, others accept that implied consent is sufficient for routine photography. Written consent is always required for photographs taken for research, audit or teaching purposes
- How will the images be stored to protect patient confidentiality?

Photographs provide good visual evidence of wound appearance. If a camera is not readily available, photography is best only considered for complicated or unusual wounds.

S = Suffering

Pain is common in patients with chronic wounds and can be either persistent (chronic) or temporary, generally related to wound care procedures (Woo *et al.*, 2008b). Pain has been discussed in Chapter 2 and pain assessment should be part of the overall patient assessment. This section will focus on local wound factors in relation to temporary pain.

An international survey of 2018 patients with chronic wounds across 15 countries identified that 21.9% had pain at dressing change 'quite often' and 31.9% had pain at dressing change 'most to all' of the time (Price *et al.*, 2008). Moreover, it took time for the pain to subside with 812 (40.2%) stating that it took less than 1 hour to resolve; for 449 (22.2%) patients it was 1–2 hours; for 192 (9.5%) patients it was 3–5 hours and for 154 (7.6%) patients it took more than 5 hours for the pain to subside. The patients were also asked what part of the dressing procedure was the most painful. They considered that touching the wound was the most painful followed by wound cleansing and dressing removal (Price *et al.*, 2008).

It is well recognised that burn patients suffer considerable pain at dressing change (Latarjet, 2002). Nagy (1999) investigated the impact on nurses of having to inflict pain on burn patients during dressing changes. She found that the commonest strategy was distancing by the nurse, which had the side-effect of the nurses becoming less concerned about controlling pain. However, if nurses developed a strategy of engaging with the pain, they saw it as a challenge to ensure good pain control. Taal *et al.* (1999) undertook a validation study of a pain anxiety scale specifically for burn patients. The scale included items such as 'I find it impossible to relax when my burns are being treated' and 'I am frightened of the pain during and/or after the treatment'. They found high levels of reliability and internal consistency and suggest that it could be used as a method of assessing therapeutic interventions.

Pain assessment has been discussed in detail in Chapter 2. Price *et al.* (2007) developed a wound pain management model that includes guidance on the assessment of wound pain and this is detailed in Figure 3.6. A comprehensive assessment will provide the basis for an effective management plan.

U = Undermining

In this part of their assessment framework Keast *et al.* (2004) discuss assessment of the internal wound area. This is relevant in cavity wounds and it is important to identify any undermining, tunnelling or sinus tracts.

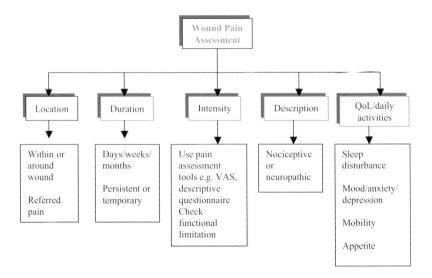

Figure 3.6 **Wound pain assessment (adapted from Wound Pain Management Model (Price *et al.*, 2007); reproduced with permission). QoL, quality of life; VAS, Visual analogue scale**

A sterile swab can be used to probe under the wound edges to measure the extent of undermining. If it is extensive it may be helpful to mark the area on the surface of the skin using a pen. This will facilitate future assessments and assist in evaluating any change.

R = Re-evaluate

The purpose of re-evaluating a wound is to check for any signs of complications and to monitor progress towards achieving short-term goals, such as debridement and the overall goal of healing. This may be achieved by checking the wound for complications such as infection at each dressing change and regularly assessing selected wound parameters such as reduction in wound size. The frequency of assessment will vary according to wound type, but for most chronic wounds it should be every 1–2 weeks. Acute wounds may need to be assessed more frequently.

In a recent review of patient outcomes, Gottrup *et al.* (2010) concluded that measuring wound reduction was valuable, but care must be taken to ensure accurate measurement of wound surface area. They considered that a 50% reduction in wound surface area over time as a useful indicator of ultimate healing. Kantor and Margolis (2000) measured percentage reduction in wound size for 104 patients with venous leg ulcers and found that percentage change in the first 4 weeks of treatment predicted the healing outcome at 24 weeks. In a small study of nine patients with grade 4 pressure ulcers, Brown (2000) found that healing did not progress in a linear fashion and suggested that plotting wound-healing curves could be useful, i.e. multiple measurements of percentage reduction in wound area from baseline, measured over time.

This type of accurate measurement may not be necessary for everyday clinical practice, but it has considerable value in research. Specialist centres may be able to invest in some of the digitised systems that can provide this type of information very easily as discussed in above but they not available to all. In general clinical practice wounds should be regularly assessed between 1 and 4 weeks as well as progress towards treatment goals evaluated.

E = Edge

This final stage of the MEASURE assessment process refers to the need to assess the wound margins and the surrounding skin. The wound margin provides useful information both indicative of aetiology and of healing status. For example, a leg ulcer with punched-out appearance and a sharp margin is indicative of an arterial ulcer. A raised edge of epithelial cells on a wound with residual slough such as can be seen in Figure 3.5 is indicative of a wound that is starting to heal; whereas Figure 3.2 shows no indication of any activity on the wound margin.

Nurses often neglect to assess the skin surrounding a wound and yet a lot of useful information can be obtained. Erythema and heat may be indicative of infection. Erythema alone may be caused by allergy to the dressing (contact dermatitis) as shown in Figure 3.7. Induration may indicate further pressure damage around an existing pressure ulcer. Maceration can occur in the presence of heavy uncontrolled exudate, if this situation persists over time, irritant dermatitis may develop (Figure 3.8). Fragile skin must be treated with caution and is at risk of damage if dressings and tapes are selected unwisely. Dry scaly skin should also be identified as scales can build up around the wound and cause problems.

Comment

Wound assessment is highly complex and is an important clinical skill. The use of uniform concepts and terms can assist in ensuring a consistent approach to the subject.

Managing wounds

A great deal has been written about wound management, but in order to make sense of what is proposed, it is helpful to understand the competing theories of wound management. These are moist wound healing and wound bed preparation.

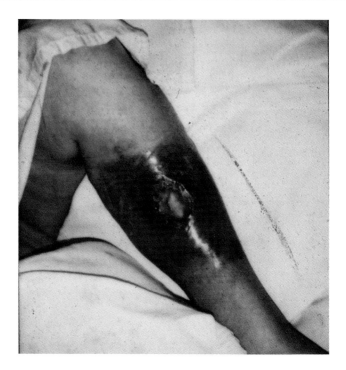

Figure 3.7   **Contact dermatitis**

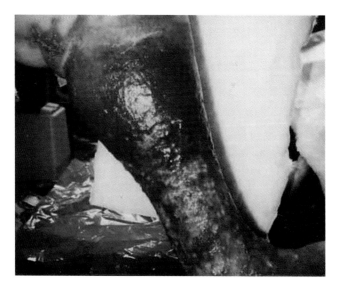

Figure 3.8   **Irritant Dermatitis**

Moist wound healing

The concept of moist wound healing was first introduced by George Winter in 1962. He compared the effect of leaving superficial wounds exposed to form a scab with that of applying a vapour-permeable film dressing, using an animal model (Winter, 1962). Epithelialisation was twice as fast in those wounds covered with a film dressing, this was because the dressing maintains humidity on the wound surface and the epithelial cells were able to slide across the surface of the wound. In contrast, epithelial cells in the exposed wounds had to burrow beneath the scab, dried exudate and layers of dessicated cells to find a moist layer to allow movement across the wound.

Little notice was taken of Winter's work until the 1980s when a number of clinical studies confirmed his findings and identified other benefits as well. Local wound pain was found to be considerably reduced in a moist environment, (May, 1984; Eaglstein, 1985; Alvarez & Dellanoy, 1987). The moist environment was also shown to enhance natural autolytic processes thus aiding the breakdown necrotic tissue (Freidman & Su, 1983; Kaufman & Hirshowitz, 1983).

Following these studies there was a dramatic change in the methods of wound management and many new occlusive wound management products have been developed such as alginates, foams, hydrocolloids and hydrogels. Schultz *et al.* (2003) summarised the benefits of a moist wound environment as follows:

- assists epidermal migration;
- promotes alterations in pH and oxygen levels;
- maintains an electrical gradient;
- retains wound fluid on the wound surface.

However, although these outcomes are of undoubted benefit to acute wounds, questions were being raised as to their usefulness in chronic wound management. Much of the research into the moist wound environment has been undertaken on acute, superficial wounds and does not address all the issues presented by chronic wounds, which tend to be deeper, with larger amounts of exudate and a greater bacterial burden. Thus a further wound management theory was required.

Wound bed preparation

The theory of wound bed preparation (WBP) has developed in part because of increasing understanding of the differences between acute and chronic wound exudate and the potentially harmful constituents of chronic wound fluid (see Chapter 1) and in part following clinical experience of using bioengineered skin products. Falanga (2000) proposed that it was

> **Box 3.1 The TIME framework (based on Falanga, 2004, reproduced by kind permission of MEP Ltd.)**
>
> **T** = Tissue Management
> **I** = Inflammation and infection control
> **M** = Moisture balance
> **E** = Epithelial (edge) advancement

inappropriate to utilise expensive, sophisticated products on a poorly prepared wound. As a minimum, a wound should have a well-vascularised wound bed, minimal bacterial burden and little or no exudate before an effective outcome can be achieved. Further debate has led to a consensus paper (Schultz *et al.*, 2003), which has provided the following definition: 'Wound bed preparation is the management of the wound to accelerate endogenous healing or to facilitate the effectiveness of other therapeutic measures'

Wound bed preparation has four aspects: debridement, management of exudate, resolution of bacterial imbalance and undermined epidermal margin (Schultz *et al.*, 2003). Falanga (2004) has utilised the work of Schultz *et al.* (2003) to develop a framework called TIME to provide a comprehensive approach to chronic wound care. The terms in the framework have been modified by the European Wound Management Association WBP Advisory Board to maximise their use in different languages (Box 3.1). Figure 3.9 shows how the TIME framework can be utilised within holistic approach to care.

Tissue management

This aspect of the TIME framework refers to the need to debride necrotic and sloughy tissue. Debridement may be achieved in a number of ways.

- Autolytic debridement utilises the ability of macrophages to phagocytose debris and necrotic tissue. Hydrocolloids and hydrogels are widely used to promote autolytc debridement as they provide a moist environment that enhances macrophage activity. Alginates are also used in the presence of moisture.
- Biosurgery or larval therapy has recently regained popularity and is widely used in the UK. Sterile maggots of the fly *Lucilia sericata* are used and they secrete enzymes that break down necrotic tissue to a semi-liquid form that the maggots can ingest, leaving only the healthy tissue (Dumville *et al.*, 2009).
- Enzymatic debridement also ensures autolysis through the use of enzymes such as elastase, collagenase and fibrinolysin. These enzymes degrade necrotic tissue and may also have an effect on fibrin, collagen

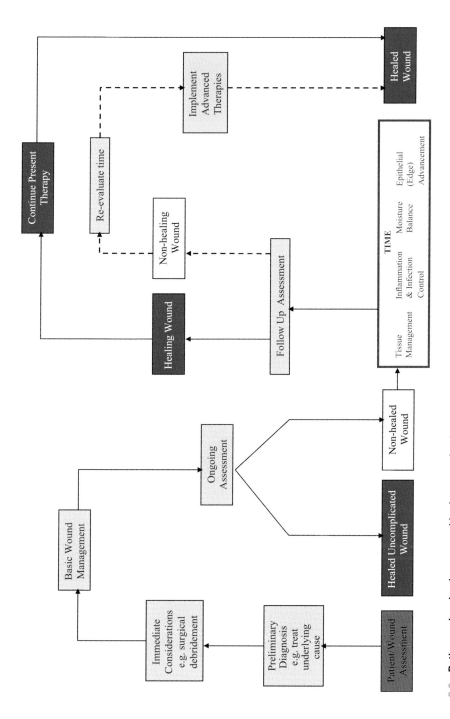

Figure 3.9 Pathway showing how wound bed preparation is applied to practice (from Falanga (2004), Reproduced by kind permission of MEP Ltd. Full document can be downloaded from www.woundsinternational.com)

and elastin (Ramundo and Gray, 2008). Although widely used in North America and mainland Europe, enzymes are rarely used in the UK.

- Mechanical debridement has been more popular in North America than elsewhere. Methods include wet-to-dry dressing, high pressure wound irrigation and whirlpool baths. Wet-to-dry dressings are saline soaked gauze swabs that are allowed to dry out and stick to the wound. They lift off slough and eschar when removed, but also cause pain to the patient and may damage newly formed tissue. There is little evidence to support their use (Cowan & Stechmiller, 2009). High-pressure irrigation can actually drive bacteria deeper into to a wound rather than washing it off. Whirlpool footbaths can potentially spread infection elsewhere on the foot and may be problematic to decontaminate between patients (Schultz *et al.*, 2003).
- Sharp or surgical debridement is the fastest method of debridement. It is of particular benefit when managing diabetic foot ulcers in preventing the build up of callus. A review by Hinchcliffe *et al.* (2008) found that although the evidence for the use of sharp debridement for diabetic foot ulcers is not strong, vigorous debridement increased the likelihood of healing at 12 weeks. However, it is not suitable for all situations. As there is potential for harm such as excessive bleeding, it should be undertaken by a competent, trained professional (Fairbairn *et al.*, 2002).

Inflammation and infection control

Chronic wounds are always colonised with bacteria but if the numbers increase then the bacterial burden increases and ultimately results in infection. The Medical Education Partnership (2008) discussed the importance of interventions to prevent further deterioration in wound with delayed healing due to increasing bacterial burden. If healing does not result from topical therapy, systemic antibiotics may be necessary, especially if a deep infection is present. Schultz *et al.* (2003) emphasise the importance of debridement as it can reduce the bacterial burden by removing devitalised tissue, a foci for bacteria, and creating a more active wound. Wolcott *et al.* (2010) also emphasise the value of debridement in removing biofilm and suggest that weekly debridement of the biofilm mass will force the biofilm to reconstitute itself. They have found the resulting immature biofilms easier to destroy. Larval therapy has also been used to reduce bacterial load and eradicate methicillin-resistant *Staphylococcus aureus* (MRSA, Dumville *et al.*, 2009). Topical antiseptics such as slow-release silver and iodine have been shown to be beneficial. However, because there are concerns about their potential toxicity, their use should be limited to reducing the bio-burden and changed to an alternative dressing once healthy granulation tissue has formed (Leaper, 2006). Topical antibiotics are not recommended because of the risk of bacterial resistance and should only be used in very specific circumstances by experienced clinicians (Medical Education Partnership Ltd, 2008).

Moisture balance

A major criticism of the moist wound healing theory is that there is no information about what constitutes the correct level of moisture on the wound surface. Wounds can produce widely varying quantities of exudate. Heavily exuding wounds may cause maceration of the surrounding skin as well as soggy dressings and a very distressed patient. On the other hand, wounds with little or no exudate may become dessicated. A balance between the two is required. The reasons for heavy exudate production should be identified and managed appropriately e.g. heavy exudate associated with infection (Okan *et al.*, 2007).

Moisture balance in the presence of heavy exudate can be achieved in a variety of ways.

- Use of highly absorbent dressings. There are a number of highly absorbent dressings available and selection depends on the type, position and size of the wound and the wound bed status. Alginates, foams and hydrofibre dressings are widely used and absorb exudate and may also have moisture vapour transmission capability. Capillary action dressings are multi-layered and able to conduct exudate away from the wound surface
- The use of appliances such as 'bag systems'. This may be by means of a stoma bag or a specialist wound appliance. These systems are only useful in wounds that constantly seep, but only contain the problem, rather than addressing it. However, they may be more effective and comfortable for the patient than bulky dressings that frequently leak (Vowden & Vowden, 2003).
- Compression is an effective method of controlling wound exudate in leg ulceration as compression reduces chronic venous hypertension. It can be achieved by the use of compression bandages or by intermittent compression therapy. This treatment is limited to leg ulcers where there is a venous component and will be discussed further in Chapter 5.
- Topical negative pressure therapy (TNP) is increasingly being applied to heavily exuding wounds of all types. A recent review by Weston (2010) summarised the effect of TNP upon the wound environment including the ability to reduce interstitial oedema; remove wound exudates and decrease bacterial colonisation.

Whatever method of moisture balance is used, it is important to care for the skin surrounding the wound. Excessive moisture can cause maceration or irritant dermatitis (Cutting & White, 2002). Various strategies may be used, depending on the method used to manage the exudate. Creams containing zinc provide an effective barrier cream and are frequently used with heavily exuding leg ulcers. They are soothing to macerated skin, but would be inappropriate where adhesive strapping is used close to the wound margin such as with TNP. Skin sealants are particularly useful under adhesive dressings as they also protect the skin from the adhesives as well as exudate. Another strategy is to use a hydrocolloid dressing, first cutting a hole the shape of the wound in the dressing wafer, and then applying it as a border around the wound as is used in biosurgery.

Epithelial (edge) advancement

A healing wound not only has a wound bed filled with healthy granulating tissue, but also evidence of epithelialisation at the wound margins. For many wounds, achieving debridement of necrosis and slough and bacterial and moisture balance will stimulate the wound to heal. However, Falanga (2004) suggests that the problems of impaired MMP metabolism or cell senescence (discussed in Chapter 1) may prevent this last phase of healing, although there is need for more research in this area. As shown in Figure 3.9, this may be the time to re-evaluate the wound and to consider the implementation of advanced therapies such as growth factors or tissue engineered products (Schultz *et al.*, 2003).

Comment

Both these theories of wound management have moved our understanding forward. It is too simplistic to suggest that moist wound healing theory should be used for the management of acute wounds and WBP for chronic wounds. Nurses should have an understanding of the underlying principles of both concepts and utilise them appropriately following a comprehensive patient and wound assessment.

Pain management

As discussed above, pain management is often neglected in wound care. Accurate assessment will determine the type and intensity of pain allowing appropriate strategies to be developed. Senecal (1999) proposed incremental steps to determine suitable analgesia and stressed the importance of regular administration. However, many patients are reluctant to take regular analgesia and may need to be encouraged to do so. Latarjet (2002) discussed the difference between background pain and procedural pain in burn patients. He considered that it is possible to achieve zero background pain, but difficult to achieve this during dressing changes. If additional medication is given before dressing change, sufficient time must be allowed for the analgesia to take effect. If pain is not controlled, it may be useful to involve the pain team.

Briggs and Torra i Bou (2002) discussed additional strategies to reduce pain. They emphasise the importance of reducing anxiety and spending time explaining to the patient what will happen and the level of pain to expect. It is also important to select appropriate dressings that will maintain moisture balance and minimise pain and trauma on removal. If dressings have adhered to the wound, then it may be necessary to soak them off. If dressings persistently adhere to the wound, an alternative dressing should be considered.

Woo *et al.* (2008a) have provided some guidance on how to minimise pain at dressing change in general as well as some statements specifically relating to dressing change.

- Cleanse wounds gently with warm saline or water. Avoid the use of abrasive wipes or cold solutions.
- Select an appropriate method of wound debridement for each wound and include the potential for causing wound-related pain.
- Select dressings that minimise trauma and pain at application and removal.

Documentation

In order to judge the progress of a wound, it is essential to keep accurate records. Good documentation will help to ensure continuity of care. Poor documentation has been implicated with frequent alterations in dressing type, according to the whim of individual nurses as shown in a study by Rundgren *et al.* (1990). They followed the progress of 101 patients with a variety of wounds over a 5-month period. They found that from week to week about 30% of the patients were receiving a different treatment. In total 65% of the wounds did not heal and patients were having treatment for the whole of the study period. They concluded that this lack of continuity was related to poor documentation, impatience and a lack of understanding of the healing process.

The European Tissue Repair Society (ETRS) have produced several statements in relation to wound management including one on documentation (ETRS, 2003). This statement is stated in full below.

- Adequate and accurate documentation of all patients with wounds should take place. This should include core information with additional information recorded depending on wound type.
- Core information should be recorded at least monthly and include:
  (a) Wound size by:
    (i) tracing;
    (ii) measurement;
    (iii) photography.

(b)   Wound bed colour (black, green, yellow, pink, red):
   (i)   % of wound bed
   (ii)   photography.
(c)   Wound depth using grading scale of initial assessment and detailing tissue at wound base.
(d)   Surrounding skin:
   (i)   healthy;
   (ii)   unhealthy.
(e)   Exudate – composition and volume:
   (i)   nil;
   (ii)   normal;
   (iii)   excessive.
(f)   Pain – continuous/dressing change/occasional.
(g)   An evaluation of treatment effect with the outcome graded as wound:
   (i)   healing;
   (ii)   static;
   (iii)   deteriorating.
(h)   The reason for non-healing indicated, e.g. infection, and the reason for treatment changes documented.

Evaluating the dressing

Nurses should be prepared to objectively evaluate the dressings they use. In particular, if they are using new dressings, although traditional dressings should not be exempt from evaluation. When evaluating a dressing, various aspects need to be considered:

- patient comfort;
- ease of application;
- effectiveness;
- cost.

Patient comfort is of primary importance for any wound management product. It can be very distressing for a patient when the application of a dressing is painful.

Some products may adhere to the wound and cause discomfort to the patients when they move and pain when the dressing is removed. A dressing that fails to provide sufficient absorbency and allows leakage of exudate, can cause considerable inconvenience, as well as promoting feelings of insecurity in the patient.

Although different nurses may carry out the dressing, the patient is always present.

Any evaluation should involve the patient. Many like to take an interest and can provide valuable information on new products.

Ease of application means that a dressing can be applied easily and so will stay in place. When using any new product, it may take a little practice to develop the most effective method of application. The nurse should be prepared to try a dressing over a period of time on a variety of wounds (unless contraindicated) and on different parts of the body. This will allow a more comprehensive evaluation.

Effectiveness is most important. If a product does not promote healing, then it does not matter if it is comfortable or easy to apply. Before a product becomes available for general use, it should have undergone stringent laboratory tests to check for safety. The ETRS (2003) has developed standards for clinical trials in wound healing that can guide the development of study protocols. Nurses may find particular difficulties undertaking a clinical trial. Hunt (1983) suggested that they included a lack of control over the admission and discharge of patients, staffing patterns and the large numbers of nurses involved in patient care and the variations in patterns of care across healthcare providers. If nurses are to evaluate the effectiveness of any dressing they use, they need to be aware of any research that has been published and any relevant systematic reviews. This will be discussed further in Chapter 7.

Cost is seen as an important factor in all aspects of care. It should be considered when evaluating any dressing. However, not only the unit cost is relevant. The overall costs should be considered. One example is a study by Thomas and Tucker (1989) who compared the use of paraffin tulle and an alginate (Sorbsan™ and found a reduced overall cost using Sorbsan™ despite the fact that the unit cost is greater than that of tulle.

References

Alvarez OM, Dellanoy OA (1987) Moist wound healing. *Paper presented at American Academy of Dermatology*.

Barber S (2008) A clinically relevant wound assessment method to monitor healing progression. *Ostomy Wound Management*, **54**: 42–9.

Bjarnsholt T, kirketerp-Møller K, Jensen PO, Madesen KG, Phipps R, Krogfelt K, Høiby N, Givskov M (2008) Why chronic wounds will not heal: a novel hypothesis. *Wound Repair & Regeneration*, **16**: 2–10.

Briggs M, Torra i Bou JE (2002) Pain at wound dressing changes: a guide to management. In: *European Wound Management Association (EWMA) Position Document: Pain at Wound Dressing Changes*. London: MEP Ltd.

Brown GS (2000) Reporting outcomes for stage IV pressure ulcer healing: a proposal. *Advances in Skin & Wound Management*, **13**: 277–283.

Browne N, Grocott P, Cowley S, Cameron J, Dealey C, Keogh A, Lovatt A, Vowden K, Vowden P (2004a) The TELER system in wound care research and post market surveillance. *EWMA Journal*, **4**: 26–32.

Browne N, Grocott P, Cowley S, Cameron J, Dealey C, Keogh A, Lovatt A, Vowden K, Vowden P (2004b) Woundcare research for appropriate products (WRAP) validation of the TELER method involving users. *International Journal of Nursing Studies*, **41**: 559–571.

Cowan LJ, Stechmiller J (2009) Prevalence of wet-to-dry dressings in wound care. *Advances in Skin & Wound Care*, **22**; 567–573.

Cutting K, Harding KG (1994) Criteria for identifying wound infection. *Journal of Wound Care*, **3**: 198–201.

Cutting K, White T (2002) Maceration of the skin and wound bed. 1 Its nature and causes. *Journal of Wound Care*, **11**: 275–278.

Davis E (1996) *Don't Deny the Chance to Heal*! Presented at: 2nd Joint Meeting of the Wound Healing Society and European Tissue Repair Society, Boston, USA, 15–19 May.

de la Brassinne M. Thirion L. Horvat LI. (2006) A novel method of comparing the healing properties of two hydrogels in chronic leg ulcers. *Journal of the European Academy of Dermatology & Venereology*, **20**: 131–5.

Dumville JC, Worthy G, Bland JM, Cullum N, Dowson C, Iglesias C, Mitchell JL, Nelson EA, Soares MO, Torgerson DJ on behalf of the VenUS II team (2009) Larval therapy for leg ulcers (VenUS II): randomised controlled trial. *BMJ*, **338**: b773.

Eaglstein WH (1985) Experiences with biosynthetic dressings. *Journal of the American Academy of Dermatology*, **12**: 434–440.

European Tissue Repair Society (2003) ETRS Working Group Statements. *ETRS Bulletin*, **10**: 10–13.

European Wound Management Association (2005) *Position Document: Identifying Criteria for Wound Infection*. London: MEP Ltd.

Fairbairn K, Grier J, Hunter C, Preece J (2002) A sharp debridement procedure devised by specialist nurses. *Journal of Wound Care*, **11**: 371–375.

Falanga V (2000) Classification for wound bed preparation and stimulation of chronic wounds. *Wound Repair and Regeneration*, **8**: 347–352.

Falanga V (2004) Wound bed preparation: science applied to practice. In: *European Wound Management Association (EWMA) Position Document Wound Bed Preparation in Practice*. London: MEP Ltd.

Flanagan M (2003) Improving accuracy of wound measurement in clinical practice. *Ostomy & Wound Management*, **49**: 28–40.

Falanga V (2004) Wound bed preparation: science applied to practice. In: European Wound Management Association (EWMA) Position Document *Wound Bed Preparation in Practice*. London: MEP Ltd.

Freidman S, Su DWP (1983) Hydrocolloid occlusive dressing management of leg ulcers. *Archives of Dermatology*, **120**: 1329–1331.

Gethin G, Cowan S (2006) Wound measurement comparing the use of acetate tracings and Visitrak™ digital planimetry. *Journal of Clinical Nursing*, **15**: 422–427.

Goldman RJ, Salcido R (2002) More than one way to measure a wound: an overview of tools and techniques. *Advances in Skin & Wound Care*, **15**: 236–243.

Gottrup F, Apelqvist J, Price P (2010) Outcomes in controlled and comparative studies on non-healing wounds: recommendations to improve the quality of evidence in wound management. *Journal of Wound Care*, **19**: 237–268.

Hack A (2003) Malodorous wounds – taking the patient's perspective into account. *Journal of Wound Care*, **12**: 319–321.

Haghpanah S, Bogie K, Wang X, Banks PG, Ho CH (2006) Reliability of electronic versus manual wound measurement techniques. *Archives of Physical Medicine & Rehabilitation*, **87**: 1396–1402.

Harding KG (1990) Wound care: putting theory into practice. In Krasner D ed. *Chronic Wound Care: A Clinical Sourcebook for Healthcare Professionals*. Malvern, PA: Health Management Publications Inc.

Hill KE, Malic S, McKee R, Rennison T, Harding KG, Williams DW, Thomas DW (2010) An *in vitro* model of chronic wound biofilms to test wound dressings and assess antimicrobial susceptibilities. *Journal of Antimicrobial Chemotherapy*, **65**: 1195–1206.

Hinchcliffe RJ, Valk GD, Apelqvist J, Armstrong DG, Bakker K, Game FL, Hartemann-Heurtier A, Löndahl M, Price PE, van Houtum WH, Jeffcoate WJ (2008) A systematic review of the effectiveness of interventions to enhance the healing of chronic ulcers of the foot in diabetes. *Diabetes/Metabolism Research & Reviews*, **24** (suppl 1): S119–S144.

Houghton PE, Kincaid CB, Campbell KE, Woodbury MG, Keast DH (2000) Photographic assessment of the appearance of chronic pressure and leg ulcers. *Ostomy & Wound Management*, **46**: 20–30.

Hunt J (1983) Product evaluation. *Nursing*, **2**: suppl. 6–7.

James GA, Swogger E, Wolcott R, Pulcini E L, Secor P, Sestrich J, Costerton JW, Stewart PS (2008) Biofilms in chronic wounds. *Wound Repair & Regeneration*, **16**: 37–44.

Jørgensen B, Bech-Thomsen N, Grenov B, Gottrup F (2006) Effect of a new silver dressing on chronic venous leg ulcers with signs of critical colonisation. *Journal of Wound Care*, 15: 97–100.

Kantor J, Margolis DJ (2000) A multicentre study of percentage change in venous leg ulcer area as a prognostic index of healing at 24 weeks. *British Journal of Dermatology*, **142**: 960–964.

Kaufman C, Hirshowitz B (1983) Treatment of chronic leg ulcers with Opsite. *Chirurgica Plastica*, **7**: 211–215.

Keast DH, Bowering CK, Evans AW, Mackean GL, Burrows C, D'Souza L (2004) MEASURE: a proposed framework for developing best practice recommendations for wound assessment. *Wound Repair & Regeneration*, **12**: supp S1–S17.

Langemo D, Anderson J, Hanson D, Hunter S, Thompson P (2008) Measuring wound length, width and area: which method? *Advances in Skin & Wound Care*, **21**: 42–45.

Latarjet J (2002) The management of pain associated with dressing changes in patients with burns. *EWMA Journal*, **2**: 5–9.

Leaper DJ (2006) Silver dressings: their role in wound management. *International Wound Journal*, **3**: 282–293.

Le Roux AA (1993) TELER the concept. *Physiotherapy*, **79**: 755–758.

McColl D, MacDougall, Medical Education Partnership Ltd (2008) Wound infection: principles of best practice. *International Wound Journal*, **5** (suppl 3): 1–11.

May SR (1984) Physiology, immunology and clinical efficacy of an adherent polyurethane wound dressing Opsite. In: Wise DL ed. *Burn Wound Coverings* (Vol. II). Boca Raton, FL: CRC Press.

McColl D, MacDougall M, Watret L, Connolly P (2009) Measuring moisture without removing the dressing. *Wounds UK*, **5**: 94–99.

Nagy S (1999) Strategies used by burn nurses to cope with the infliction of pain on patients. *Journal of Advanced Nursing*, **29**: 1427–1433.

Okan D, Woo K, Ayello EA, Sibbald RG (2007) The role of moisture balance in wound healing. *Advances in Skin & Wound Care*, **20**: 39–53.

Papazoglou ES, Zubkov L, Mao X, Nidrauer M, Rannou N, Weingarten MS (2010) Image analysis of chronic wounds for determining surface area. *Wound Repair & Regeneration*, **18**: 349–358.

Price P, Fogh K, Glynn C, Krasner DL, Osterbrink J, Sibbald RG (2007) Managing painful chronic wounds: The wound pain management model. *International Wound Journal*, **4** (suppl 1): 4–15.

Price PE, Fagervik-Morton H, Mudge EJ, Beele H, Ruiz JC, Nyström TH, Lindholm C, Maume S, Melby-Østergaard B, Peter Y, Romanelli M, Seppänen S, Serena TE, Sibbald G, Soriano JV, White W, Wollina W, Woo KY, Wyndham-White C, Harding KG (2008) Dressing-related pain in patients with chronic wounds: an international patient perspective. *International Wound Journal*, **5**: 159–171.

Ramundo J, Gray M (2008) Enzymatic wound debridement. *Journal of Wound, Ostomy and Continence Nursing*, **35**: 273–280.

Rundgren A, Nordehammar A, Bjornestol A, Magnusson H, Nelson C (1990) Pressure sores in hospitalised geriatric patients. Background factors, treatment, long-term follow-up. *Care - Science and Practice*, **8**: 100–103.

Schultz GS, Sibbald RG, Falanga V, Ayello EA, Dowsett C, Harding K, Romanelli M, Stacey MC, Teot L, Vanscheidt W (2003) Wound bed preparation: a systematic approach to wound management. *Wound Repair and Regeneration*, **11** (suppl): S1–S28.

Senecal S (1999) Pain management of wound care. *Nursing Clinics of North America*, **34**: 847–860.

Shaw J, Hughes CM, Lagan KM, Bell PM, Stevenson MR (2007) An evaluation of three wound measurement techniques in diabetic foot wounds. *Diabetes Care*, **30**: 2641–2642.

Sibbald RG, Meaume S, Kirsner RS, Münter KC (2006) Review of the clinical RCT evidence and cost-effectiveness data of a sustained-release silver foam dressing in the healing of critically colonised wounds. *World Wide Wounds* (http://www.worldwidewounds.com).

Stremitzer S, Wild T, Hoelzenbein T (2007) How precise is the evaluation of chronic wounds by health care professionals? *International Wound Journal*, **4**: 156–161.

Sugama J, Sanada H, Konya C, Okuwa M, Kitagawa A (2007) A study of the efficiency and convenience of an advanced portable wound measurement system (Visitrak™). *Journal of Clinical Nursing*, **16**: 1265–1269.

Taal LA, Faber AW, van Loey NEE, Reynders CLL, Hofland HWC (1999) The abbreviated burn specific pain anxiety scale: a multicentre study. *Burns*, **25**: 493–497.

Thomas S, Tucker CA (1989) Sorbsan in the management of leg ulcers. *Pharmaceutical Journal*, **243**: 706–709.

Van Pouche S, Vander Haeghen Y, Vissers K, Meert T, Jorens P (2010) Automatic colorimetric calibration of human wounds. *BMC Medical Imaging*, **10**: 7 (http://www.biomedcentral.com/1471-2342/10/7).

Vowden K, Vowden P (2003) Understanding exudate management and the role of exudate in the healing process. *British Journal of Nursing*, **12** (suppl): 4–13.

Weston C (2010) The science behind topical negative pressure therapy. *Acta Chirugia Belgica*, **110**: 19–27.

Werdin F, Tennenhaus M, Schaller H-E, Rennekampff H-O (2009) Evidence-based management strategies for treatment of chronic wounds. *Eplasty*, **9**: e19.

White RJ (2006) Critical colonisation – the concept under scrutiny. *Ostomy Wound Management*, **52**: 50–56.

Winter GD (1962) Formation of the scab and the rate of epithelialisation of superficial wounds in the skin of the domestic pig. *Nature*, **193**: 293.

Wolcott RD, Rumbaugh KP, James G, Schultz G, Phillips P, Yang Q, Watters C, Stewart PS, Dowd SE (2010) Biofilm maturity studies indicate sharp debridement opens a time- dependent therapeutic window. *Journal of Wound Care*, **19**: 320–328.

Woo KY, Harding K, Price P, Sibbald G (2008a) Minimising wound-related pain at dressing change: evidence-informed practice. *International Wound Journal*, **5**: 144–157.

Woo KY, Sibbald G, Fogh K, Glynn C, Krasner D, Leaper D, Österbrink J, Price P, Teot L (2008b) Assessment and management of persistent (chronic) and total wound pain. *International Wound Journal*, **5**: 205–215.

World Union of Wound Healing Societies (2007) *Principles of Best Practice: Wound Exudate and the Role of Dressings. A Consensus Document*. London: MEP.

Wound Management Products

Introduction

There are many wound management products available and considerable conflicting advice on how they should be used. Many nurses have a great interest in this subject. They take a justifiable pride in the acquired skills that facilitate dressing change. Recent developments have demonstrated a need to change or adapt traditional practices.

Wound management products include topical agents as well as dressings and also what has been described as 'advanced dressings'. A topical agent is that which is applied to a wound. A dressing is a covering on a wound that is intended to promote healing and protect from further injury. Advanced products are much more sophisticated dressings compared to those in everyday usage. The Department of Health divides dressings into primary and secondary. A primary dressing is used in direct contact with the wound. A secondary dressing is superimposed over the primary dressing. The use of all these products will be discussed in this chapter.

The development of dressings through the ages

In *L'Ingenu* (1767/1978) Voltaire described history as a 'tableau of crimes and misfortunes'. A study of the dressings used through the ages suggests that there may be some truth in this. Some of the treatments used on the wounded were bizarre, if not horrific, whereas others are still familiar today.

Early days

The earliest record of any dressing can be found on the Edwin Smith Papyrus. Edwin Smith was an American Egyptologist who bought the papyrus from a trader in Luxor in 1862. He was unable to translate it and its contents were unknown until a complete translation was published in 1930

The Care of Wounds: A Guide for Nurses, Fourth Edition. Carol Dealey.
© 2012 Carol Dealey. Published 2012 by John Wiley & Sons, Ltd.

(Zimmerman & Veith, 1961). The papyrus is dated at around 1700 BC, but it is a copy of original manuscripts that date back to around 3000–2500 BC. A variety of dressings are mentioned including grease, honey, lint and fresh meat, which was valued for its haemostatic properties. Adhesive strapping was made by applying gum to strips of linen (Forrest, 1982)

As the power of Ancient Egypt waned, the Greek civilisation gradually developed. Amongst the men who made their mark at this time was Hippocrates. He lived from about 460–377 BC. Hippocrates laid the basis for scientific medicine with his emphasis on careful observation. For the most part, Hippocrates considered that wounds should be kept clean and dry. He recommended tepid water, wine and vinegar for cleansing wounds. If a wound showed signs of inflammation, he suggested applying a cataplasm or poultice to the area around the wound to soften the tissues and to allow free drainage of pus (Zimmerman & Veith, 1961). Hippocrates also used propolis, a hard resinous material produced by bees, to help in the healing of sores and ulcers (Trevelyn, 1997). Hippocrates gave the first definition of healing by first intention, where the skin edges are held in approximation to each other, and secondary intention where there is tissue loss and the skin edges are far apart.

Some of these concepts can also be found in the writings of Sushruta. He was an Indian surgeon who lived sometime between the sixth century BC and the sixth century AD. His surgical textbook the *Sushruta Samhita* has been used as a basis for later writers. Sushruta described 14 different types of dressings made from silk, linen, wool and cotton (Zimmerman & Veith, 1961). He also placed great emphasis on the importance of cleanliness. Meade (1968) describes Sushruta's recommendations for the management of wounds involving the intestines. First black ants were applied and then the intestines were washed in milk and lubricated with clarified butter before they were returned to their normal position. He differed from Hippocrates on the matter of the most appropriate diet for patients. Sushruta considered meat, normally forbidden to Hindus, an important factor, whereas Hippocrates recommended the restriction of food and gave his patients only water to drink. (Zimmerman & Veith, 1961).

The influence of Greek physicians continued on into the time of the Roman Empire. Oil and wine were commonly applied to wounds. Reference to this was made by the Gospel-writer Luke, when he was recording the parable of the Good Samaritan. Luke describes the Good Samaritan pouring oil and wine onto the wounds and then applying bandages.

Celsus compiled a history of the development of medicine from the time of Hippocrates to the first century AD with great detail of the practices of his time. Although it is believed that Celsus was not a physician, he was the first to give a definition of inflammation. He listed the cardinal signs as redness, heat, pain and swelling. He advocated the cleansing of wounds to remove foreign bodies before suturing. He also expected wounds to suppurate, that is, to form pus (Meade, 1968). A Roman scholar, Pliny, described the use of propolis (bee's wax) to soften induration and reduce swelling. He also wrote that it healed sores when healing seemed impossible (Trevelyn, 1997).

It is, however, Galen who stands out as the person whose work had lasting impact. Galen (AD 129–199) worked as the surgeon to the gladiators in Pergamun and later as physician to the Emperor Marcus Aurelius. He wrote many books, some of which survived him and were seen as the ultimate in medical knowledge for many centuries. He is particularly known for his theory of laudable pus ('pus bonem et laudabile'). This theory holds that the development of pus is necessary for healing and should, therefore, actively be promoted. Galen found the application of writing ink, cobwebs and Lemnian clay to wounds to be efficacious (Forrest, 1982). When reviewing his achievements, Duin and Sutcliffe (1992) considered that although in some ways Galen considerably expanded medical knowledge, he also held it back for a thousand years.

The dark age and early middle ages

After the fall of the Roman Empire, cultural influence moved eastwards and the Arab doctors of Islam further developed medical knowledge. However, their wound care was based on Galenic teaching. A number of doctors, such as Rhazes and Albucassis, translated Galen's writings into Arabic, but the most famous was Ali Ibn Al-Husain-al-Sina (980–1037). He was also known as Avicenna to the Western World. Avicenna wrote the *Canon Medicina*, translating Galen's work and adding his own commentary (Dealey, 2002). Ultimately it was translated into both Hebrew and Latin and became seen as the foremost medical textbook in the Middle East, North Africa and Europe up until the seventeenth century (Guthrie, 1945). Avicenna proposed treating pressure ulcers with white lead ointment, covering the bed with salix leaves and preventing the patient from sleeping on his back (Kanal, 1975). He also advised the use of astringents such as cooked honey and myrrh to reduce the amount of exudate in wounds with tissue loss.

Medical knowledge swept across the Middle East, through North Africa and into Spain and Southern Italy with the spread of Islam and the Islamic Empire. Thus the teaching of the Arab doctors influenced many of the developments in Europe including reinforcing the pre-eminence of Galen. It must also be recognised that during this time the Church supplied most of the healthcare provision outside the home, resulting in the Church having control over many aspects of medicine, such as giving support to Galenic teaching.

Salerno, in southern Italy was the first European university to have a medical school, which was founded in the ninth century (Forrest, 1982). Unlike most other universities of the time, Salerno was not under ecclesiastical control and so was able to incorporate surgery into the curriculum as a time when the clergy were prohibited from practising it (Zimmerman &

Veith, 1961). Salerno was the leading centre for surgical training in the eleventh century and during this time the *Surgery of Roger* was written. It was translated into 15 other languages and was used up to the sixteenth century (Paterson, 1988). Roger advocated the use of lard in head wounds, either applied directly or soaking cloth in molten lard for deep wounds. He did not recommend cleaning wounds, but used dressings made from eggs and water, tow and salt and bandages of fine linen cloth (Paterson, 1988).

One of the expert surgeons who graduated from Salerno was Hugo of Lucca (1160–1257). He went on to found the School of Surgery at Bologna University (Dealey, 2003). Although none of his writings have survived, he was considered to be a very innovative surgeon. His famous pupil, Theodoric (also known at Teodrico Borgognoni) (1205–?1296) completed his *Chirurgia* or surgical textbook in 1267, which he stated was based on Hugo's teaching. Theodoric disagreed with the concept of laudable pus as he considered that it prolonged healing. He advocated cleaning a wound with wine, debriding it and removing all foreign matter, approximating the wound edges and holding them in place using compresses of lint soaked in warm wine and then binding them in place. The dressing was then to be left *in situ* for 5–6 days, unless there was excessive heat or pain (Borgognoni, 1955). He proposed that chronic wounds should be cleansed with honey mixed with wine and water of holm oak or vine ashes; alternatively, seawater could be used to cleanse and dry a wound. Unfortunately, his work was discredited and gradually his ideas disappeared until the twentieth century when it was re-discovered in Italy (Popp, 1995)

One of the people influenced by Theodoric's teaching was Henri de Mondeville (1260–1320). He was a French doctor who trained in Paris and Montpellier as a physician, before going to Bologna to learn surgery from Theodoric (Gerster, 1910). He was highly respected as a man of profound erudition and moral character and became surgeon to King Phillippe le Bel of France in 1301. De Mondeville also wrote a *Chirurgie*, which drew on the work of Avicenna for anatomy and Theodoric for wounds. Unfortunately, de Mondeville was not a tactful person and he commenced his treatise on wounds by first describing and then condemning the common practices of the day that promoted laudable pus. Unsurprisingly, he failed to influence his contemporaries who tried to put pressure on him to abandon his treatment (Dealey, 2004).

A close successor to de Mondeville was Guy de Chauliac (1300-1368). He followed a similar training pattern to de Mondeville, training in Toulouse, Montpellier and Paris before travelling to Bologna to study anatomy (Johnson, 1989). It was when de Chauliac was in Bologna that he became strongly influenced by Galen's writing. This is reflected in his *Grande Chirurgie* in which he quoted Galen 890 times (Johnson, 1989). When writing about wound care he rejected the ideas of Theodoric and de Mondeville and proposed treatments such as the use of tents (drains) and meshes (packing) to hold wounds open and oily salves to promote pus formation.

De Chauliac's book was highly successful, having numerous editions and translations and it became the primary surgical textbook for 200 years. He had so great an influence that his critics consider that he set back progress in wound management for up to six centuries, although not every commentator takes such a harsh view (Johnson, 1989).

Late middle ages and renaissance

Kirkpatrick and Naylor (1997) have described the contents of a surgical treatise dated 1446 and believed to be the work of Thomas Morstede (1380–1450) who was a London surgeon. The work provides detailed information about the classification of ulcers and their treatment. The step-by-step approach describes how to enlarge the mouth of the ulcer, then the processes of mortification (debridement), mundification (cleansing) and fleshing (encouragement of granulation tissue). The recipes for the various topical applications are provided for the reader. They include items such as sage leaves, wormwood, white Gascony wine, alum and honey for mundification. The recipe for a treatment for fleshing involved stirring the mixture for the length of time it took to say two creeds.

Ambroise Paré (1510–1590) was the most famous surgeon of the Renaissance period (Zimmerman & Veith, 1961). He rose from a poor background with little education to become surgeon to four successive French kings, ultimately gaining the title *Premier Chirurgien* and *Conseiller du Roi*. However, it is as a military surgeon that Paré is best known. With the discovery of gunpowder, warfare changed. Gunshot wounds were believed to be poisonous. In order to treat them, surgeons began to undertake more amputations of limbs. The standard practice was to use boiling oil to cauterise the stump. Paré is famous for using a mixture of egg yolks, oil of roses and turpentine instead. Paré is also well known for his saying 'Je le pensait, Dieu le guarist', which is generally translated as 'I dressed him, God healed him' (Zimmerman and Veith, 1961). Paré proposed using a dressing composed of rock alum, verdigris, Roman vitriol, rose honey and vinegar, boiled together to form a paste on traumatic wounds (Linker & Womack, 1969). He treated a severe pressure ulcer by encouraging the patient, feeding him, providing pain relief and sleep-inducing medication and pressure relief by means of a small pillow (Levine, 1992). Paré wrote numerous books, all in the vernacular rather than Latin. Some of his later writings are considered to be classics.

The seventeenth, eighteenth and early nineteenth centuries

The first book entirely about burns was published in 1614. It was called *De Combustionibus* and written by Wilhelm Fabry a German wound surgeon. The book was translated into English by Kirkpatrick *et al.* (1995) and they considered that it contained a number of original ideas and observations with a lot of practical advice on the management of burns. Fabry discussed burn injury and described three degrees of severity, a term used until recently. He included sections on pain management and the importance of sleep and rest as well as the management of scars and contractures. Fabry also described in detail some of the wound dressings he used, for example an ointment of raw onions, salt, white and blue soap, rose oil and sweet almond oil to treat first degree burns (Kirkpatrick *et al.*, 1995).

Another doctor worthy of mention is the German surgeon, Lorenz Heister (1683–1758). Heister was exceeding well educated in languages and the humanities as well as medicine and surgery at a time when most of his colleagues had little education or training and charlatans abounded (Zimmerman & Veith, 1961). He developed his skills working as a military surgeon and became a professor of anatomy and surgery at the University of Helmstadt in 1719. He wrote a general system of surgery in three parts: the doctrine and management of (I) wounds of all kinds, (II) several operations; and (III) bandages (Heister, 1768). Heister used lint dressings made up in various formats such as dipped in alcohol or oil of turpentine to treat haemorrhage or spread with a sound digestive ointment or balsam to heal wounds. He suggested that wound edges should not closed, in order to allow pus to drain. He believed that all bandages should be made from clean linen that had been softened by repeated use (Bishop, 1959). His book was translated into numerous languages including English and ran to 10 editions.

Many of the developments in wound management seem to be associated with wounds from battles. One development was that of debridement, possibly originated by Henri Francois LeDran (1685–1770) in order to relieve the constriction of soft tissues, believed to be caused by inflammation following gunshot wounds (Helling & Daon, 1998). However, other surgeons across Europe suggested caution in its use. John Hunter (1728–1793), the famous English surgeon disagreed with the practice as he did not believe that wounds should be made larger in order to remove extraneous matter. He thought that suppuration would bring it to the surface (Zimmerman & Veith, 1961). During the Napoleonic wars, several French surgeons advocated the use of debridement, particularly in the care of gunshot wounds (Helling & Daon, 1998). However, its use was sporadic and most wounds were not explored and after the fall of Napoleon and his empire the concept was almost entirely forgotten.

Mid-Nineteenth and early twentieth century developments

The Crimean War led to a huge demand for dressings. Various types of dressings were produced in the workhouses, which were a source of cheap labour. Charpie was made from unravelled cloth. Oakum was old rope, which had been unpicked and teased into fluff, it became popular with doctors during the American Civil War as they considered it to be very absorbent (Bishop, 1959). Tow was made from broken, ravelled flax fibres. Lint is linen that has been scraped on one side. The production of this dressing was mechanised. All of these dressings were washed and re-used many times. They gradually became quite soft, but they were not very absorbent.

Sheets of cotton wool retained by cotton bandages were used during the Franco–Prussian wars, but Joseph Sampson Gamgee (1828–1886) was the person who further developed its use. He noted that cotton wool could be made absorbent by removing the oily matter within it. He then conceived the idea of covering the cotton wool with unbleached gauze to make dressing pads or gamgee tissue (Lawrence, 1987). Gamgee tissue is still available today.

In 1867, Lister introduced the use of carbolic acid and revolutionised surgery and surgical wound management. When he realised that carbolic caused skin irritation, he developed a method of impregnated carbolic gauze that became the first antiseptic dressing (Bishop, 1959). The use of antiseptics and concept of asepsis spread rapidly across Europe.

During the course of the World War I, more and more severely wounded soldiers had to wait several days before receiving more than a simple field dressing. As a result, many wounds became infected and gangrenous. Antiseptics were developed to help resolve this problem. In particular, two similar antiseptic solutions came into use. They were Eusol (Edinburgh University Solution of Lime) and Dakin's solution. Other antiseptics such as iodine, carbolic acid and mercury and aluminium chloride were also available.

Sinclair and Ryan (1993) have reviewed some of the medical literature of 1915 to identify thinking at that time on the use of antiseptics. Bond (1915) considered that it was important to apply a 'germicide' as early as possible to wounds that were almost certain to be infected. British soldiers were advised to carry tincture of iodine so that they could apply it immediately to any gunshot wounds (Mayo-Robson, 1915). However, Herzog (1915) writing of the German experience in the battlefield reported that he had seen a number of soldiers suffering from dermatitis of the skin around the wound as a result of the indiscriminate use of iodine.

Deparge, a Belgian surgeon of note, recognised that merely introducing antiseptics into war wounds was insufficient and he re-introduced the concept of wound debridement (Helling & Daon, 1998). He believed that such devastating wounds, often covered in mud and dirt and receiving only minimal surgery encouraged the development of soft tissue infections. He developed a set of principles for managing them that involved exploring the wound and excision of all contaminated and contused tissue, followed by leaving the wound open and irrigating it with Dakin's solution. He also favoured the use of delayed primary closure or secondary closure if bacteria were present. Deparge's use of debridement has had a major impact on trauma surgery (Helling & Daon, 1998).

At this time, Lumiere devised a dressing called tulle gras, a gauze impregnated with paraffin. Sphagnum moss was also used as it was found to be twice as absorbent as cotton wool. It could also be impregnated with antiseptics and sterilised. Eupad was a dressing designed for use on leg ulcers. It was a Eusol preparation, made up with a mixture of boracic and bleach. Another popular type of dressing was Emplastrums. These were made of white leather spread with a plaster mass, to which some type of medication was often added (Turner, 1986).

During World War II an American neurosurgeon called Eldridge Camp-bell was with a field hospital in Italy. In 1943 there was a great deal of heavy fighting and many casualties. Some of the Italian doctors who were involved in caring for these patients proposed a method of wound care that involving cleansing and debriding the wound and then suturing it. This was contrary to current practice of the day, which recommended packing with vaseline gauze and immobilisation. Campbell was impressed by this method of healing and eventually traced its origins back to the thirteenth century and Theodoric. In describing this fascinating piece of medical history, Popp (1995) concludes that it demonstrates the problems of entrenched views that are not questioned such as the teachings of Galen and the dangers of summarily dismissing new ideas.

The British Pharmaceutical Codices

The first British Pharmaceutical Codex was published in 1907. It provided information on all the drugs and medicinal preparations in common use throughout the British Empire. Turner (1986) has reviewed the dressings listed in the earliest British Pharmaceutical Codices and compared them with more recent lists of dressings in the British Pharmacopoeia. He found that the list from 1923 contains much that is familiar today. Gauzes, cotton wool pads and bandages can be seen as very popular methods of wound care. Turner suggests that it is only in the last 30 years that any attempt has been made to design materials that are actually functional. Prior to that, dressings were made from materials that happened to come to hand.

Traditional techniques

Today nurses expect to perform the vast majority of dressings, other than simple first aid treatments applied in the home or workplace. But this was not always the case. Originally, dressings changes were undertaken by doctors. Eventually, medical students, particularly on surgical wards were trained to change dressings. By the 1930s, the task was given to experienced sisters. Ultimately, it became a recognised nursing task.

During the 1930s and 1940s, as the care of wounds gradually came into the nursing domain, much mystique became attached to the subject. This was exaggerated with the development of an aseptic, usually non-touch, technique. Merchant (1988) has reviewed the literature on this subject and concluded that the procedure that was developed in the 1940s was still being used at the time she was writing, despite the change to a central sterile supply system. Most hospitals had changed to this system by the early 1970s.

In the early days, large water sterilisers were used for preparing the equipment for an aseptic procedure. One was usually found on every ward. It was the task of the night nurses to boil all the metal bowls, receivers and gallipots, ready for the morning dressing round. The dressings were packed in drums and sent to a central point for sterilising. It was left to the ward sister to choose what went into the drum. Commonly, gauze squares, cotton wool balls and wadding were used. In many hospitals nurses wore masks and gowns, a practice that gradually disappeared. Usually two nurses carried out the dressing, a clean nurse and a dirty nurse. Much attention was paid to the position of the equipment on top of the trolley and to the frequency and timing of hand washing.

All wounds were redressed once or twice daily. The wound was thoroughly cleaned using cotton wool balls and forceps. The method of wiping across the wound surface varied from hospital to hospital. The Hippocratic principle of keeping wounds clean and dry became adapted to 'allowing wounds to dry up'. Mostly gauze preparations were used, but gradually all sorts of dubious practices crept in. There have been reports of Marmite, eggs and even toast being used on wounds (Dobrzanski *et al.*, 1983; Johnson, 1987).

A wide variety of pharmaceutical preparations have also been applied without any recognition of the need for evidence-based care. Several studies have shown the wide range of dressings being used in different areas. Murray (1988) found that within her health authority an amazing selection of pharmaceutical products were in use: 18 different cleansing agents, 53 substances left in contact with open wounds and 24 products used for packing wounds. Millward (1989) found 19 different substances being used on pressure ulcers within one hospital. Walsh and Ford (1989) discussed the rituals being used in nursing at that time, much of which could be applied to wound care. The common reasons for choosing a dressing could be listed as:

- we always do it that way here;
- Sister said so;
- I have used this dressing for the last 30 years, why should I change?

Many nurses will have been trained to use these ritualistic methods. It is only recently that there has been a critical evaluation of these methods and changes made to a more evidence-based approach.

The use of lotions

A variety of lotions are used in wound care, primarily for wound cleansing. The aims of wound cleansing are to remove any foreign matter such as gravel or soil, to remove any loose surface debris such as necrotic tissue and to remove any remnants of the previous dressing. A systematic review by the Joanna Briggs Institute (2008) did not find any evidence to either support or refute the practice of swabbing or scrubbing wounds in order to cleanse them. Bee *et al.* (2009) undertook a similar systematic review and found that using an irrigation pressure for 5–8 psi there was a significant reduction in the wound bioburden (this can be achieved using a 35 ml syringe and a 19 G needle.) Several reviews have found that potable tap water can safely be used as an alternative to normal saline (e.g. Joanna Briggs Institute, 2008; Bee *et al.*, 2009; Fernandez *et al.*, 2010). Cutting (2010) has discussed the use of tap water as a cleanser in the light of the problem of biofilms (see Chapter 3). He suggested that although the choice of cleansing solution should be based on the requirements of a specific wound, tap water or normal saline may not be the optimal choice for all and there is probably still a role for some antiseptics.

Antiseptics

After saline, the commonest type of lotion in use is an antiseptic. An antiseptic can be defined as a non-toxic disinfectant, which can be applied to skin or living tissues and has the ability to destroy vegetative compounds, such as bacteria, by preventing their growth. If they are simply used to wipe across the wound surface they will have little effect. Antiseptics need to be in contact with bacteria for about 20 minutes before they actually destroy them (Russell *et al.*, 1982). In some instances they can be applied in the form of soaks or incorporated into dressings, ointments or creams.

Research using experimental wounds in the animal model has demonstrated antiseptics have toxic effects that need to be weighed against any advantages obtained from their use. In the late 1980s and early 1990s there was considerable debate about the use of antiseptics and their widespread use has dramatically reduced. Since the introduction of the concept of wound bed preparation (discussed in Chapter 3), antiseptics have made somewhat of a come back as they are seen to have a place in achieving bacterial balance (Schultz *et al.*, 2003). A review by White *et al.* (2006) suggested that although there needs to be judicious use of antiseptics, their use may be preferable to the use of antibiotics in relation to bacterial resistance. Lipsky and Hoey (2009) suggest that it is safer to use antiseptics in modern formats rather than solutions as they seem to be less toxic. However, they also conclude that, in the light of the limited evidence for their use, antiseptics should be used very selectively and for a short time only.

The following section on antiseptics is divided into two parts, those which are still commonly used and those which are rarely used and have little evidence to support their use.

Widely used antiseptics

Iodine

Iodine is a broad-spectrum antiseptic and is available as an alcohol and an aqueous solution. The aqueous solution is used in wound care, usually as povidone iodine 10%, which contains 1% available iodine. It is used as a skin disinfectant and to clean grossly infected wounds. McLure and Gordon (1992) and Michel and Zach (1997) found it to be effective against meth-icillin-resistant *Staphylococcus aureus* (MRSA). Several studies have questioned the value of using povidone iodine. It is cytotoxic to fibroblasts unless diluted to 0.001%, retards epithelialisation and lowers the tensile strength of the wound (Lineaweaver *et al.*, 1985). Brennan and Leaper (1985) found that povidone iodine 5% damaged the microcirculation of the healing wound, but a 1% solution was innocuous. In contrast, Bennett *et al.* (2001) found that povidone iodine significantly increased fibroblast proliferation, and slightly increased neodermal regeneration and epithelialisation.

Povidone iodine has been used within the wound bed preparation model of wound management. Wilson *et al.* (2005) found povidone iodine 10% to be highly toxic to keratinocytes. In a review of its use by Leaper and Durani (2008) the authors concluded that, although there are limitations in the evidence available, it is a useful antiseptic that is less toxic than others substances such as chlorhexidine or silver sulphadiazine. Povidone iodine is available in ointment, spray and powder form and impregnated into dressings.

Cadexemer iodine is a form of slow-release iodine incorporated into a dressing. It retains antibacterial properties and is effective against common pathogens found in chronic wounds as well as having the ability to destroy biofilms (Leaper & Durani, 2008; Hill *et al.*, 2010). It has been widely used on chronic wounds and, although there are limitations in the quality of the research, it would seem to be effective reducing wound infection and increasing healing rates (Leaper & Durani, 2008).

Iodine should not be used for patients with thyroid disease or who have are sensitive to the product.

Silver

Silver has been used as an antiseptic in wound care for many years in the form of silver nitrate. However, it is extremely caustic, stains the skin black and prolonged use causes hyponatraemia, hypokalaemia and hypocalcaemia. To overcome these problems a cream, silver sulphadiazine, was developed and has been very successful in controlling burn wound infections (Lansdown, 2004). However, the combination of cream and exudate means dressing removal can be messy and is usually undertaken in a hydrotherapy unit, which can be a source of cross-infection (Tredget *et al.*, 1998). As a result, there is increasing interest in the use of silver-coated dressings of varying types.

Wright *et al.* (1998) tested the bacteriacidal effect of silver in three modalities: liquid (silver nitrate), cream (silver sulphadiazine) and a silver-coated dressing. All products were effective at killing bacteria. The silver-coated dressing was the most efficacious against a wider range of bacteria and silver nitrate the least efficacious. Silver has been incorporated into a number of modern wound management dressings. A large pragmatic randomised trial of silver dressings versus standard care in venous leg ulcers found no difference in healing rates (Michaels *et al.*, 2009). However, it should be noted that there was no attempt to identify wound infections or the level of the bioburden in these wounds. The important conclusion from the study is that silver dressings are more expensive to use than standard dressings and should not be used as an alternative to standard dressings. However, this does not mean they are not effective in managing infected wounds.

Silver dressings will be discussed in more detail below.

Honey

Honey has been used in wound care since ancient times and there has been a recent resurgence of interest in its use, particularly manuka honey (Flanagan, 2000). Honey is listed here as it has antimicrobial properties. The high sugar content creates an osmotic effect drawing exudate and bacteria from the wound (Sharp, 2009). Honey also has a low pH, which creates an environment that is inhospitable to bacteria. Honey has been shown to be effective against most common wound-infecting bacteria and MRSA and vancomycin-resistant enterococci (Wijesinghe *et al.*, 2009). Honey dressings come in a variety of formats and will be discussed in more detail below.

Polyhexamethylene biguanide

Polyhexamethylene biguanide (PHMB) is used widely as a sanitiser and disinfectant. It is also used as a wound cleanser in USA and mainland Europe, but is less well known in the UK (Wounds UK, 2010). Recently it has been incorporated into several dressings. When used as a wound cleansing fluid it is generally used combined with betaine. Betaine has a surfactant effect and helps to remove debris from the wound surface. Phillips *et al.* (2010) suggest that the betaine component reduces surface tension on the wound surface, thus promoting cleansing and may be particularly beneficial in removing biofilms.

In a German study, retrospective analysis was undertaken of 112 patients with chronic leg ulcers. They found a reduced infection rate in the group whose wounds were cleansed with PHMB/betaine compared with the group who had saline and Ringer's solution (Kaehn & Eberlein, 2008). A retrospective study of venous leg ulcer patients compared 59 patients treated with PHMB with 53 patients whose ulcers were cleansed with a combination of saline and Ringer's solution (Andriessen and Eberlein, 2008). They found the incidence of wound infection was 3% ($n = 2$) in the PHMB group compared with 13% ($n = 7$) in the control group. It should also be noted that there was a statistically faster healing time for the PHMB group than the control (3.31 months compared with 4.42 months; $p = <0.0001$).

Rarely used antiseptics

Cetrimide
Cetrimide is useful for its detergent properties, particularly for the initial cleansing of traumatic wounds or the removal of scabs and crusts in skin disease. It should not be used in contact with the eye. It is rapidly inactivated by organic material. Two dangers should be noted, it can cause skin irritation and sensitivity, and, it is very easy for it to become contaminated by bacteria, especially *Pseudomonas aeruginosa*. It is rarely used and not available in the USA (Lipsky & Hoey 2009).

Chlorhexidine
Chlorhexidine is used in a variety of aqueous formulations. It is effective against Gram-positive and Gram-negative organisms. Brennan *et al.* (1986) found that it has a low toxicity to living cells. Tatnall *et al.* (1990) undertook a similar study to identify the toxicity of several antiseptics when used on cultured keratinocytes (used for grafts). They found chlorhexidine to be the least toxic, but considered that antiseptics should not be used over these graft sites. Kearney *et al.* (1988) found that it could maintain its antimicrobial levels for a period of time when impregnated into a dressing. However, the efficacy of chlorhexidine is rapidly diminished in the presence of organic material such as pus or blood (Reynolds, 1982). Mengistu *et al.* (1999) tested chlorhexidine in different strengths against a range of Gram-negative bacteria and found that a significant number were only inhibited by high concentrations of chlorhexidine. They concluded that it was more suitable for disinfection and hospital hygiene rather than wound care.

Hydrogen peroxide 3%
Hydrogen peroxide 3% (10 vols) has an oxidising effect that destroys anaerobic bacteria. However, it loses its effect when it comes in contact with organic material such as pus or cotton gauze. Lineaweaver *et al.* (1985) showed that hydrogen peroxide was cytotoxic to fibroblasts unless diluted to a strength of 0.003%. This dilution is not effective against bacteria. O'Toole *et al.* (1996) found that even in concentrations 1000-fold less than 3% dilution it inhibits keratinocyte migration and proliferation. Bennett *et al.* (2001) found that 3% hydrogen peroxide significantly reduced neodermal regeneration and fibroblast proliferation compared to controls

(untreated wounds) in an animal model study. There is also a report of an incident where an air embolism occurred after irrigation with hydrogen peroxide (Sleigh and Linter, 1985). Rees (2003) reviewed the evidence on hydrogen peroxide and concluded that it was unsuitable for use in cleaning wounds in A&E. Hydrogen peroxide is no longer widely used, there is no evidence to demonstrate its efficacy and there are a number of other more suitable alternatives.

Potassium permanganate 0.01%

Potassium permanganate 0.01% is mostly used on heavily exuding eczematous skin conditions, generally associated with leg ulceration. It is most easily used in the form of tablets. One tablet dissolved in 4 litres of water provides a 0.01% solution.

The affected limb is generally placed in a container holding the fluid for approximately 15 minutes. It is mildly deodorising and has slight disinfectant properties. It has been found to cause staining of the skin. There is little evidence to demonstrate its efficacy (Anderson, 2003).

Proflavine

Proflavine has a mild bacteriostatic effect on Gram-positive organisms, but not on Gram-negative bacteria. There has been little research to demonstrate its value. Although it is available as a lotion it is mostly used as an aqueous cream. However, proflavine is not released from the cream into the wound, so has no effect on the bacteria. Foster and Moore (1997) compared the use of proflavine-soaked gauze packs with cellulose-based fibre dressing in surgical cavity wounds. They found that the proflavine packs were significantly more painful to remove and patients required analgesia prior to removal.

Sodium hypochlorite

Sodium hypochlorite comes in several forms, the commonest being Eusol, Dakin's Solution and Milton. It was originally used on heavily infected wounds during the World War I. Dakin suggested that for it to be effective, it should be used in large volumes, (Thomas, 1990). Several research studies have been undertaken that suggest that the hypochlorites may have little beneficial effects and do much harm.

It is cytotoxic to fibroblasts, unless diluted to a strength of 0.0005%, and retards epithelialisation, (Lineaweaver *et al.*, 1985). Brennan and Leaper (1985) found that it caused considerable damage to the microcirculation of the wound. Wilson *et al.* (2005) found modified Dakin's solution was highly toxic to keratinocytes. Bennett *et al.* (2001) found that half-strength sodium hypochlorate had a mixed effect on wound repair, with no impairment of fibroblast proliferation but decreased vascular density. However, at that strength it was ineffective as an antimicrobial.

Carneiro and Nyawawa (2003) randomly allocated Eusol or phenytoin powder to treat 102 leg ulcers. They found that there was a significant reduction in pain, exudate levels and wound size in the phenytoin group compared with the Eusol group. This study was undertaken in Tanzania and many of the ulcers were due to animal bites. These ulcers were found to heal fastest. The authors concluded that phenytoin was a more suitable than Eusol, especially as it is cheap and easily applied.

Another study in a tropical country compared Eusol with honey for the treatment of surgical cavity wounds following the drainage of abscesses in 32 children in Nigeria (Okeniyi *et al.*, 2005). The researchers found significantly faster healing and reduction of hospital stay in the honey group and concluded that it was a superior product. On the whole, the use of Eusol and other hypochlorates is now obsolete.

Antibiotics

A range of antibiotics is available in topical form. They are potentially hazardous and they are not always absorbed into the wound. Medical Education Partnership (2008) stated that it is best to avoid the use of topical antibiotics in order to minimise the risk of allergy and bacterial resistance. Systemic antibiotics are the treatment of choice when treating infected wounds because the infection may be too deep for topical antibiotics to penetrate. However, they may not be effective against biofilms (Rhoads *et al.*, 2008). An *in vitro* study using a model for biofilms in chronic wounds found that two commonly used antibiotics (flucloxacillin and ciprofloxacin) were ineffective against the biofilm in the model (Hill *et al.*, 2010).

One preparation which would seem to be of benefit in wound care is mupirocin. Mupirocin is used predominantly for treating MRSA either in skin infections or for the nasal colonisation. Several studies have demonstrated its efficacy in treating MRSA in burn wounds (Rode *et al.*, 1989; Deng *et al.*, 1995; Trilla and Miro, 1995). Erdur *et al.* (2008) found mupirocin effective against *S. aureus* in experimental crush wounds. However, the guidelines for the prophylaxis and treatment of MRSA warn that there is increasing resistance to mupirocin and recommend that it should only be used in conjunction with systemic antibiotics (Gemmell *et al.*, 2006).

Saline 0.9%

This is the only completely safe cleansing agent and is the treatment of choice for use on most wounds. Manufacturers recommend that it is used in conjunction with many of the modern wound management products. Saline is presented in sachets, small plastic containers that allow the saline to be squirted onto the wound and also in aerosols. These last two presentations are more widely used in the community.

Tap water

> Tap water is being used more frequently on a variety of wounds. In particular, on areas already colonised such as wounds following rectal surgery or leg ulcers. Many patients may bath or shower prior to dressing change. There seems to be little point in then 'cleansing' the wound. However, the bath or shower should be thoroughly cleaned afterwards to avoid cross-infection. A recent systematic review found that there is no evidence that using tap water to cleanse acute wound increases infection rates (Fernandez *et al.*, 2008). It would therefore seem reasonable to suggest that either saline or water may be used, selection being based on practicality and individual circumstances.

Clinically effective wound management products

> Originally dressings were seen merely as coverings that could provide some protection to the wound. The range of products currently available for use is much more sophisticated. There are so many products to choose from that it can cause considerable confusion. There is no single perfect dressing but an 'identikit' list of criteria can be established. The requirements of a specific wound may not need all of the criteria listed. Selection can be assisted if the nurse has:

> - assessed the wound and identified the specific objectives for the wound at that time;
> - an understanding of what can be reasonably expected from a dressing
> - access to information regarding the characteristics and effectiveness of the range of dressings available to the nurse.

> The characteristics of a clinically effective wound management product will be considered below. Dressings are generally considered in relation to their performance and their handling qualities. Performance relates the ability to promote healing.

Providing an effective environment

> The qualities that will promote an effective environment for healing were discussed in Chapter 3 under theories of wound management. They are:

> - ability to maintain a moist environment;
> - antibacterial properties;
> - fluid handling properties;

These qualities can be listed as:

- easy to apply;
- conformability;
- easy to remove;
- comfortable to 'wear'
- does not require frequent dressing change.

Easy to apply

A major advantage of many of the modern products is that they are very simple and quick to apply. Realistically, this has helped to promote their use with the nurses who regularly provide wound care.

Conformability

A dressing that conforms well to the shape of the wound is likely to assist in maintaining a moist environment and also provide an effective barrier for bacteria.

Easy to remove

If a dressing is easy to remove it is less likely to damage any of the newly formed tissue in the wound. It is also less likely to be painful for the patient.

Comfortable to 'wear'

Another advantage of many modern products is that they are comfortable for the patient when they are *in situ*. This means that the patient is more likely to want to comply with the treatment regime. In any case, there is no need for patients to suffer unnecessary pain or discomfort.

Does not require frequent dressing change

The majority of modern products can be left in place for several days, depending on the wound and, particularly, the amount of exudate. This not only saves nursing time and reduces costs but also reduces the amount of interference with the wound. Reduction in the frequency of dressing change helps to reduce the opportunities for a drop of temperature on the wound surface. This can potentially occur at each dressing change. Myers (1982) studied 420 patients and found that, after wound cleansing, it was 40 minutes before the wound regained its original temperature. Furthermore, he found that it took 3 hours for mitotic activity to return to its normal rate. Patients also find less frequent dressing changes beneficial. Some patients find dressing change an ordeal and others, especially community patients, an inconvenience that disrupts their life.

Comment

It should be recognised that no one dressing provides the optimum environment for the healing of all wounds and it may be necessary to use more than one type of dressing during the healing of a wound. Many dressings will fulfil some of the criteria and they should be selected following careful assessment of the wound. (See Chapter 3.)

Modern wound management products

In order to make sense of all the dressings that are available, they will be divided into different categories. Dressings can also be considered in terms of their suitability as a primary or secondary dressing on open wounds. In the UK, not all the dressings are freely available in the community as government restrictions control which dressings can be prescribed. This may considerably affect continuity and quality of care between hospital and community.

The categories used in the UK *Nurse Prescribers' Formulary* (BMJ Group & RPS Publishing, 2009) are used as a template. Readers wishing to find information about details about proprietary products may refer to the *Nurse Prescribers' Formulary* or at www.dressings.org.

Basic wound contact dressings

Low-Adherent dressings

These types of dressing are low adherent rather than non-adherent. They have little if any absorbent capacity and are best on wounds with little exudate. They mostly need to be used in combination with an absorbent pad. They do not provide a moist wound environment. Examples of this type of dressing are *knitted viscose dressings* and *tulle dressings*. Tulles are also called paraffin gauze and were originally known as tulle gras. They are made of open-weave cotton or rayon impregnated with soft paraffin. Although the paraffin makes the dressing less adherent, it readily becomes incorporated into granulation tissue. A pattern can be seen on the wound surface when it is removed. They do not maintain a moist wound environment and have no absorbent capacity.

Absorbent dressings

The dressings described in this section have variable levels of absorbency.

Absorbent perforated dressings with adhesive border
These dressings consist of a central pad, which is covered with a wider band of adhesive backing. They are lightweight and usually remain in position

satisfactorily. There is little absorbent capacity in these dressings. They are widely used on post-surgical wounds, which are healing by first intention, but are not suitable for open wounds as a primary dressing.

Absorbent perforated plastic-film faced dressing
These are low-adherent dressings, generally of three layers. They have little absorbency. There are many dressings available in this category.

Absorbent cellulose dressings with fluid-repellent backing
They are one-piece multilayer dressings that are highly absorbent and able to wick exudate away from the wound surface. They may be used in direct contact with the wound and are intended for use on heavily exuding wounds of all types.

Advanced dressings

Advanced dressings are now widely used in the developed world and their use is spreading. They are listed in order of their absorbent capacity, starting with those with low absorbency

Hydrogels

These dressings are made from insoluble polymers and have a high water content. They have the ability to either absorb exudate or hydrate dry wounds such as necrotic eschar, thus encouraging debridement. They all require a secondary dressing.

Hydrogel sheets
The gel sheets are best used on granulating moderate to low exuding wounds. They are not suitable for infected wounds.

Hydrogel application (amorphous)
The amorphous gel may be used on a wide variety of wounds. They can be used on wounds with moderate to low exudate and in small cavities.

Vapour-permeable films and membranes

Film dressings allow the passage of moisture vapour through the film but do not allow the passage of water or organisms. They provide a moist healing environment but have no absorbency. They should not be used on infected wounds.

Vapour-permeable adhesive film dressing
The method of application of these film dressings varies according to make. Most require a certain amount of skill and practice in application.

Vapour-permeable adhesive film dressing with absorbent pad
These dressings have been developed to address the fact that film dressings have no absorbency. They can be used on wounds with low exudate.

Soft-polymer dressings

Many of the soft-polymer dressings contain silicone and have been developed to provide gentle adhesive properties. This ensures that they can be removed easily from fragile skin, reducing pain and trauma. Suitable for wounds with moderate to low exudate, these dressings may be covered with an outer pad or have their own integral pad.

Hydrocolloid dressings

Hydrocolloids are a development from stoma products. They are interactive dressings consisting of a hydrocolloid base made from cellulose, gelatins and pectins and a backing made from a polyurethane film or foam. Hydrocolloid dressings come in several different formats: with and without a border, a hydrocolloid fibrous dressing and a polyurethane matrix dressing. They also come in a wide range of sizes and shapes and variations such as one thinner than the standard dressing. No secondary dressing is necessary.

Hydrocolloid dressing without adhesive border
There are a number of these dressings that may have variable levels of capacity to absorb exudate.

Hydrocolloid dressing with adhesive border
The adhesive border is intended to assist in dressing retention over awkward areas of the body.

Hydrocolloid-fibrous dressings
These dressings are made from hydrocolloid fibres that gel in the presence of exudate. They are highly absorbent and present as a flat dressing in a range of sizes and also a ribbon for cavity wounds. They are not suitable for use over dry necrotic wounds.

Polyurethane-matrix dressing
These dressings are made from a polyurethane matrix with absorbent particles and an outer polyurethane film cover.

Foam dressings

Foam dressings are made from polyurethane foam and are best used on granulating or epithelialising wounds with some exudate. They come in a number of formats. *Polyurethane foam film dressings with or without adhesive border* are suitable for wounds with low to moderated exudate as they have a low absorbent capacity whereas *polyurethane foam dressings* and *polyurethane foam dressings with adhesive border* have greater absorbency. They are available in a variety of shapes and sizes. Foam dressings are also available for cavity wounds either as a pre-formed foam stent or as a version that has to be mixed with a catalyst and then poured into the wound cavity where it sets in the shape of the wound.

Alginates

Alginate dressings contain calcium or sodium alginate, which is derived from seaweed. This type of dressing is an interactive dressing because as it reacts with the wound its structure alters. As the dressing absorbs exudate it changes from a fibrous structure to a gel. Some dressings allow removal in one piece, others have to be flushed from the wound. These dressings are available in a variety of formats, flat dressings, rope or ribbon, extra-absorbent versions and with an adhesive backing. They are appropriate for moderate or heavily exuding wounds and may require a secondary dressing. They should not be used on wounds with no or low exudate.

Capillary action dressings

These dressings are non-interactive three-layered dressings made from hydrophilic filaments sandwiched between two low-adherent wound contact layers. They absorb exudate into the middle layer and wick it laterally in a capillary action. They may be cut to shape to fit a cavity and are suitable for all types of heavily exuding wounds. However, capillary-action dressings are contraindicated for heavily bleeding wounds or arterial bleeding.

Odour-Absorbent dressings

This group of dressings contain activated charcoal that can absorb wound odour. Some versions may be more suitable as a secondary dressing and others are a combination of charcoal and an advanced dressing and so can be used as a primary dressing. It should be noted that the primary goal for malodorous wounds is to reduce or remove the factors that contribute to the odour. Charcoal dressings can be useful until that goal is achieved.

Antimicrobial dressings

Antiseptics and antimicrobials have been discussed in some detail above. This section will describe the various formats of dressings containing antimicrobials.

Honey

The commonest type of honey used in wound care is Manuka honey, but South African and Bulgarian honey are also available. Medical-grade honey has become very popular in recent years and so has been incorporated into a number of different dressing types. *Sheet dressings* range from knitted viscose or tulles to alginate or hydrogel dressings, impregnated with honey. It is also available as a *honey-based topical application* when the honey is supplied in tubes ready to be squeezed into the wound.

Iodine

There are dressings available that incorporate povidone iodine or cadexemer iodine into their structure. Povidone iodine is impregnated into a knitted viscose dressing. It is suitable for superficial wounds with low to moderate exudate as the iodine is rapidly deactivated in the presence of exudate. Cadexemer iodine dressings are composed of hydrophilic beads containing iodine. As they absorb exudate, the beads swell and gel and the iodine is released slowly into the wound. They come in the form of a powder or an ointment. This dressing is intended for heavily exuding necrotic, sloughy or infected wounds. It should not be used for more than 3 months at a time and is not suitable for people with iodine sensitivity or thyroid problems.

Silver

In recent years silver has been overused and it has been incorporated into most types of advanced dressings: low-adherence dressings; with charcoal; soft polymer dressings; hydrocolloid dressings; foam dressings and alginate dressings. It is recommended that silver dressings should only be used when there is known or suspected wound infection (BMJ Group & RPS Publishing, 2009).

Specialised dressings

Protease-modulating dressings

These dressings have the ability to alter the activity of matrix metalloproteinases (MMPs) in chronic wounds. As yet there is limited evidence to demonstrate whether this approach has any clinical significance.

Silicone keloid dressings

Silicone gel and gel sheets are used to help with scar management as they are able to soften and flatten keloid and hypertrophic scars. The sheets can be washed and reused. They are not suitable for open wounds.

Skin protection

Barrier-film dressings

Barrier-film dressings have been developed to protect the skin. Some films were originally developed for use around stoma sites. The film is wiped on using an applicator such as an impregnated towel or sprayed on and dries to form a film barrier protecting the skin from adhesives as well as moisture and they are resistant to urine and faeces.

Complex adjunct therapies

Biosurgery

Biosurgery is another name for maggot or larvae therapy. The use, often inadvertent, of maggots in wounds has been recognised for centuries. Morgan (1995) chronicled the use of maggots from Maya Indians through to the 1930s. He considered that the use of maggots fell into disrepute with the advent of antibiotics and aseptic wound care. He also noted the aesthetic problems with their usage. However, the use of larvae therapy is enjoying a resurgence of popularity at present. Thomas *et al.* (1996) suggest this return in popularity might be in part because of the problems caused by resistant bacteria such as MRSA.

The larvae for biosurgery are supplied in sterile containers directly from the supplier. They may be 'free range' within a small plastic container or sealed within a porous bag. Before applying the larvae, a hydrocolloid dressing should be applied around the wound to protect the skin from the proteolytic enzymes produced by the maggots (Sherman, 1997). Once placed in the wound, the free-range maggots are retained by means of a small net, taped in place; those in a bag are simply placed in the wound and held in place with tape. Once the larvae are removed from the wound, they are disposed of in the same way as all used dressings. They are used to debride necrotic, sloughy and infected tissue from a wound.

A randomised, controlled trial by Dumville *et al.* (2009) compared loose or bagged larvae and a hydrogel for the treatment of sloughy or necrotic leg ulcers. There was no difference in outcome between the two types of larvae and in time to healing between the three groups. However, the larvae were found to debride the leg ulcers faster than the hydrogel.

Topical negative pressure therapy

Topical negative pressure (TNP) therapy is a device that applies a universal negative pressure to a wound encouraging blood flow and faster granulation (Baxandall, 1996). There are now several TNP products that either use foam or gauze as the wound-contact layer. Tubing connects the wound to the pump via a canister to collect exudate. The wound contact layer and the end of the tubing are covered with a film dressing to create an airtight seal. Pressure can be applied continuously or intermittently.

Argenta pioneered the development of TNP therapy. He described successful outcomes in 296 of 300 cases of chronic, acute and subacute wounds that they treated (Argenta and Morykwas, 1997). Subsequently, there have been numerous reports of its use, many of which have been case series or case studies.

Several systematic reviews of TNP have been undertaken and the two most recent are reported here. Ubbink *et al.* (2008) undertook a Cochrane review of the use of TNP for both acute and chronic wounds and included 15 randomised, controlled trials of variable quality in the review. They found that the use of TNP did not speed healing times in chronic wounds but did reduce the time needed to prepare acute wounds for secondary closure. The reviewers overall conclusion was that there is little evidence to support the use of TNP in wound management. Wasiak and Cleland (2007) undertook a Cochrane review of TNP for partial-thickness burns in 2007 that was updated in 2010. They drew a similar conclusion to Ubbink *et al.* (2008) that there is little evidence to support the use of TNP. Despite these very negative reviews, TNP is very widely used, particularly on complex or non-healing acute wounds.

Two guidance documents on the use of TNP have been produced by two separate panels of international experts. The first (Bovill *et al.*, 2008) was by a group of surgeons, most of whom were plastic surgeons and the second (Bollero *et al.*, 2010) a group of surgeons, physicians and nurses. There was no overlap between the two groups of experts. In both instances the guidance was based on the available evidence of laboratory studies, case series and clinical trials as well as the panel members own clinical experience. Some of the guidance pertains to surgical procedures and so is beyond the remit of this book, but the more general guidance is considered here. Bollero *et al.* (2010) suggest that TNP is not the most appropriate choice for all wounds and suggest that although it might be the product of choice in some situations, it should be considered on a patient-by-patient basis for others.

When to use TNP

- In deep cavity wounds to stimulate granulation.
- To manage high levels of exudate.
- To prepare the wound bed for grafting.
- To reduce bioburden – it should be noted that although TNP is widely used for this purpose, there is evidence that it does not actually reduce bacterial load (Braakenburg *et al.*, 2006; Mouës *et al.*, 2004).

When not to use TNP

- When the wound is covered with necrotic eschar.
- Exposed vital organs present.

- Untreated osteomyelitis close to the wound.
- Malignancy in the wound.
- Active bleeding or risk of bleeding in the wound.
- Allergies to any of the components of TNP.

When to stop using TNP
TNP should be discontinued if:

- the goals of treatment have been achieved;
- there is failure to improve and the wound deteriorates or infection worsens;
- complications such as excessive bleeding develop;
- poor patient compliance or the patient is unable to tolerate the therapy.

Little research has been undertaken into the patients' perspective of TNP. A recent qualitative study (Abbotts, 2010) undertook a mixture of focus groups and interviews with 12 patients who had experience of TNP. Analysis of the transcripts identified a number of themes. The participants were positive about the therapy as they considered it healed their wounds faster. However, most of them were bothered by the smell of malodorous exudate coming from the canister and some were embarrassed by the tubing and pump. Pain was also a factor for some patients, especially at dressing change. Some of the patients had been discharged home with TNP and although they struggled with the dressing changes they seemed to manage general activities of daily living. It was generally agreed that there was a lack of written patient information and they recommended that something should be made available.

It is obvious that whilst TNP is widely used, more high-quality research is required in order to provide the evidence that is required to underpin its use.

Hyperbaric oxygen

Hyperbaric oxygen chambers have been used for many years for recompression therapy for divers with the bends or decompression illness. More recently it has also been used for non-healing wounds. Hyperbaric oxygen (HBO) treatment has been defined as 'the patient breathing in 100% oxygen intermittently at a point higher than sea level pressure' (British Medical Association Board of Science and Education, 1993). It is delivered by placing a patient inside a pressure chamber, which may be designed for one or more people. The length of time over which treatments are given varies according to the condition being treated.

Sander *et al.* (2009) investigated the effects of HBO therapy on non-impaired and impaired wound healing using an animal model, in particular studying the effect on angiogenesis and epithelialisation. They found that it significantly speeded up the rate of epithelialisation in both non-impaired and impaired wounds compared with those not treated with HBO. They also found the same significant result when assessing rates of angiogenesis.

Kranke *et al.* (2004) undertook a Cochrane review of five randomised studies using HBO. Four of the studies were of diabetic foot ulcers (a total of 147 patients). The authors were able to pool the results of three studies and found a reduction in the risk of major amputation with HBO therapy compared with controls. A numbers-needed-to-treat analysis showed that four patients would need to be treated in order to prevent one amputation in the long term. Kranke *et al.* (2004) also reviewed a study of 16 venous ulcer patients. Although there was a significant reduction in ulcer size in the HBO group, the numbers are very small. They conclude that overall, the reviewed studies were of poor quality and inadequately reported. There seems to be a benefit for diabetic foot ulcers, but there is a need for adequately powered, randomised studies that include an economic evaluation. This review was revisited in 2009 and the authors concluded that the results remained the same. More recently a randomised, controlled trial was undertaken comparing HBO with placebo for 94 patients with diabetic foot ulcers (Löndahl *et al.*, 2010). They found significantly greater numbers of healed ulcers in those patients who received <35 HBO treatments compared with placebo.

Hyperbaric oxygen is also used for acute surgical and traumatic wounds and this was the subject of a recent Cochrane review (Eskes *et al.*, 2010). The authors only found three studies suitable for inclusion in the review. They found the studies to be small and of poor quality with a high risk of bias. They concluded that although there is a suggestion that HBO may improve outcomes for skin grafts and traumatic wounds, this must be treated with caution because of the risk of bias.

It is obvious that there is only a limited case for the use of hyperbaric oxygen at present. However, for most nurses the argument is academic as they are not likely to have access to such equipment.

Tissue culture

Tissue culture describes the process whereby a small full-thickness section of skin is harvested from a patient or donor and then cultured in the laboratory to form large sheets of cells (cultured keratinocytes). The sheets of cells are then grafted onto a granulating wound that is completely free of any necrotic material. Autologous tissue (that is, taken from the patient) has been found to be more effective than allogenic tissue (that is, taken from a donor). Tissue culture has become well established since the early1980s when the first clinical reports of its use appeared.

Lee *et al.* (2009) discussed the development of multi-layered cell structures called three-dimensional freeform fabrication and described how they used it to create a multilayered culture of human skin fibroblasts and keratinocytes. The computer used within the fabrication could potentially be used to create wound-specific skin layers that would 'match' the surrounding skin. However, this work needs testing on wound models before it can be applied clinically.

On the whole, cultured keratinocytes have been used by plastic surgeons particularly for treating burn patients. Tissue culture is an important therapy for burn patients. It may have potential for wider use, but needs some further development.

Tissue engineering

Tissue engineering takes tissue culture a step forward. It uses human dermal fibroblasts and cultures them on a biosynthetic scaffold. The fibroblasts proliferate and secrete proteins and growth factors resulting in the generation of a three-dimensional human dermis that can then be used to graft over wound sites. Two brands are currently available: Apligraf® (also known as Graftskin) and Dermagraft®. Their construction is slightly different. Apligraf® is an allogeneic bi-layered cultured skin equivalent whereas Dermagraft® is a human fibroblast-derived dermal substitute

Two large multi-centre, multinational randomised studies of Apligraf® have been undertaken in USA, Europe and Australia to determine the effect of Apligraf® on non-infected neuropathic diabetic foot ulcers (Veves *et al.*, 2001; Edmonds *et al.*, 2009). All patients had surgical debridement prior to treatment and adequate foot off-loading. Both studies found a significantly faster rate of healing at 12 weeks compared with the standard treatment of saline-moistened gauze. Marston *et al.* (2003) undertook a similar study comparing Dermagraft® with conventional treatment for diabetic foot ulcers of greater than 6 weeks duration and also found a significantly faster rate of healing at 12 weeks in the Dermagraft® group.

Falanga *et al.* (1998) studied the effect of using Apligraf® on patients with venous ulcers in a multicentre trial. A total of 240 patients were randomised to Apligraf® and compression or compression therapy alone. They found a significantly faster healing rate in the Apligraf® group. In those patients ($n = 120$) whose ulcer had been open for more than year, Apligraf® was significantly more effective in achieving healing.

Omar *et al.* (2004) undertook a pilot study using Dermagraft® for venous ulcers. Eighteen patients were randomised to either the Dermagraft® and compression or compression alone and followed-up for 12 weeks. Five patients in the Dermagraft® group and one of the control's ulcers were healed at 12 weeks, but this did not achieve significance. However, there was a significant reduction in ulcer size and in the linear rate of healing in the Dermagraft® group.

Allenet *et al.* (2000) used a Markov model to undertake an economic evaluation of the costs of using Dermagraft® compared with standard treatment for diabetic foot ulcers over a 52-week period. The overall treatment costs were lower for Dermagraft® because of a faster healing rate (53,522FF compared with 56,687FF). Redekop *et al.* (2003) undertook a similar exercise comparing Apligraf® with general wound care for diabetic foot ulcers. They found that there was a 12% reduction in costs using Apligraf®.

It would seem that the use of human skin equivalents has considerable potential in the treatment of wounds that have failed to heal after utilising other methods. Although the economic evaluations described above indicate that cost savings can be made using them, it should be remembered that this is only the case in those wounds that are not healing. Other methods should be used first, before considering human skin equivalents.

References

Abbotts J (2010) Patients' views on topical negative pressure: 'effective but smelly'. *British Journal of Nursing*, **19** (suppl.): S37–S41.

Allenet B, Paree F, Lebrun T, Carr L, Posnett J, Martini J, Yvon C (2000) Cost-effectiveness modelling of Dermagraft for the treatment of diabetic foot ulcers in the French context. *Diabetes & Metabolism*, **26**: 125–132.

Anderson I (2003) Should potassium permanganate be used in wounds? *Nursing Times*, **99** (suppl): 19.

Andriessen A, Eberlein T (2008) Assessment of a wound cleansing solution in the treatment of problem wounds. *Wounds*, **20**: 171–175.

Argenta LC, Morykwas MJ (1997) Vacuum-assisted closure: a new method for wound control and treatment: clinical experience. *Annals of Plastic Surgery*, **38**: 563–576.

Baxandall T (1996) Healing cavity wounds with negative pressure. *Nursing Standard*, **11**: 49–51.

Bee TS, Maniya S, Fang ZR, Yoong GLN, Abdullah M, Choo JCN, Towle RM, Hong WY, Gaik ITC (2009) Wound bed preparation - cleansing techniques and solutions: a systematic review. *Singapore Nursing Journal*, **36**: 16–21.

Bennett LL, Rosenblum RS, Perlov C, Davidson JM, Barton RM, Nannet LB (2001) An in vivo comparison of topical agents in wound repair. *Plastic and Reconstructive Surgery*, **108**: 675–685.

Bishop WJ (1959) *A History of Surgical Dressings*. Chesterfield: Robinson and Sons Ltd.

BMJ Group & RPS Publishing (2009) *Nurse Prescribers' Formulary 2009-2011*. London: BMJ Group & RPS Publishing.

Bollero D, Driver V, Glat P, Gupta S, Lazaro-Martinez JL, Lyder C, Ottonello M, PelhamF, Vig S, Woo K (2010) The role of negative pressure wound therapy in the spectrum of wound healing. *Ostomy Wound Management*, **56** (suppl): 1–18.

Bond, CJ (1915) The application of strong antiseptics to wounds. *British Medical Journal*, **March 6**: 405–406.

Borgognoni T (1955) *The Surgery of Theodoric* (vol. 1) (translated from the Latin by Campbell E, Colton J). New York: Appleton-Century-Crofts Inc.

Bovill E, Banwell PE, Teot L, Eriksson E, Song C, Mahoney J, Gustafsson R, Horch R, Deva A, Whitworth I (2008) Topical negative pressure wound therapy: a review of its role and guidelines for its use in the management of acute wounds. *International Wound Journal*, **5**: 511–529.

Braakenburg A, Obdeijn MC, van Rooij IALM, van Griethuysen AJ, Klinkenbijl JHG (2006) The clinical efficacy and cost-effectiveness of the vacuum-assisted closure technique in the management of acute and chronic wounds: a randomised controlled trial. *Plastic & Reconstructive Surgery*, **118**: 390–397.

Brennan SS, Leaper DJ (1985) The effect of antiseptics on the healing wound: a study using the rabbit ear chamber. *British Journal of Surgery*, **72**: 780–782.

Brennan SS, Foster ME, Leaper DJ, (1986) Antiseptic toxicity in wounds healing by second intention. *Journal of Hospital Infection*, **8**: 263–267.

British Medical Association Board of Science and Education (1993) *Clinical Hyperbaric Medicine Facilities in the UK*. London: British Medical Association.

Carneiro PM, Nyawawa ET (2003) Topical phenytoin versus EUSOL in the treatment of non-malignant leg ulcers. *East African Medical Journal*, **80**: 124–129.

Cutting K (2010) Addressing the challenge of wound cleansing in the modern era. *British Journal of Nursing*, **19**: S24–S29.

Dealey C (2002) Wound healing in Moorish Spain. *EWMA Journal*, **2**: 32–34.

Dealey C (2003) Wound healing in medieval and renaissance Italy: was it art or science? *EWMA Journal*, **3**: 15–17.

Dealey C (2004) The contribution of French surgeons to wound healing in medieval and renaissance Europe. *EWMA Journal*, **4**: 33–35.

Deng S, Sang J, Cao L (1995) The effects of mupirocin on burn wounds with staphylococcus aureous infection. *Chung Hua Cheng Hsing Shao Shang Wai Ko Tsa Chih*, **11**: 45–48.

Dobrzanski, S., Duncan,S.E., Harkiss,A., Ball,A. and Robertson,D. (1983) Topical applications in pressure sore therapy. *British Journal of Pharmaceutical Practice*, **5**: 10.

Duin N, Sutcliffe J (1992) *A History of Medicine*. London: Simon & Schuster.

Dumville JC, Worthy G, O Soares M, Bland JM, Cullum N, Dowson C, Iglesias C, McCaughan D. Mitchell JL, Nelson EA, Torgerson DJ (2009) VenUS II: a randomised controlled trial of larval therapy in the management of leg ulcers. *Health Technology Assessment*, **13**: 1–182.

Edmonds M and European and Australian Apligraf Diabetic Foot Ulcer Study Group (2009) Apligraf in the treatment of neuropathic diabetic foot ulcers. *International Journal of Lower Extemity Wounds*, **8**: 11–18.

Erdur B, Ersoy G, Yilmaz O, Ozcuturk A, Sis B, Karcioglu O, Parlak I, Ayrik C, Aksay E, Guruay M (2008) A comparison of the prophylactic uses of topical mupirocin and nitrofurazone in murine crush contaminated wounds. *American Journal of Emergency Medicine*, **26**: 137–143.

Eskes A, Ubbink DT, Lubbers M, Lucas C, Vermeulen H (2010) Hyperbaric oxygen therapy for treating acute surgical and traumatic wounds. *Cochrane Database of Systematic Reviews*, **10**: CD008059.

Falanga V, Marolis D, Alvarez O, Auletta M, Maggiocomo F, Altman M, Jensen J, Sabolinski M, Hardin-Young, J. (1998) Rapid healing of venous ulcers and lack of clinical rejection with an allogeneic cultured human skin equivalent. *Archives of Dermatology*, **134**: 293–300.

Fernandez R, Griffiths R (2008) Water for wound cleansing. *Cochrane Database of Systematic Reviews*, **1**: CD003861.

Flanagan M (2000) Honey and the management of infected wounds. *Journal of Wound Care*, **9**: 287.

Forrest RD (1982) Early history of wound treatment. *Journal of the Royal Society of Medicine*, **75**: 198–205.

Foster L, Moore P (1997) The application of a cellulose-based fibre dressing in surgical wounds. *Journal of Wound Care*, **6**: 469–473.

Gemmell CG, Edwards DI, Fraise AP, Gould FK, Ridgeway GL, Warren RE (2006) Guidelines for the prophylaxis and treatment of MRSA infections in the UK. *Journal of Antimicrobial Chemotherapy*, **57**: 589–608.

Gerster AG (1910) Surgical manners and customs in the times of Henry de Mondeville. *Proceedings of the Charaka Club*, **3**: 70–90.

Guthrie D (1945) *A History of Medicine*. London: Thomas Nelson & Sons Ltd.

Heister L (1768) A *General System of Surgery in Three Parts*, 6th edn. (translated into English by Heister LJ). London: Whiston.

Helling TS, Daon E (1998) In Flanders fields: the Great War, Antoine Deparge and the resurgence of debridement. *Annals of Surgery*, **228**: 173–181.

Herzog, W. (1915) German experiences. The dangers of tincture of iodine as a first-aid dressing. *British Medical Journal*, **March 6**: 441–442.

Hill KE, Malic S, McKee R, Rennison T, Harding KG, Williams DW, Thomas DW (2010) An in vitro model of chronic wound biofilms to test dressings and assess antimicrobial susceptibilities. *Journal of Antimicrobial Chemotherapy*, **65**: 1195–1206.

Lawrence JC (1987) A century after Gamgee. *Burns*, **13**: 77–79.

Joanna Briggs Institute (2008) Solutions, techniques and pressure in wound cleansing. *Nursing Standard*, **22**: 35–39.

Johnson A (1987) Wound Care, packing cavity wounds. *Nursing Times*, **83**: 59–62.

Johnson PC (1989) Guy de Chauliac and the Grand Surgery. *Surgery, Gynaecology and Obstetrics*, **169**: 172–176.

Kaehn K, Eberlein T (2008) Polyhexanide (PHMB) and Betaine in wound care management. *EWMA Journal*, **8**: 13–17.

Kanal H (1975) *Encyclopaedia of Islamic Medicine*. Cairo: General Egyptian Book Organisation.

Kearney JN, Arain T, Holland KT (1988) Antimicrobial properties of antiseptic impregnated dressings. *Journal of Hospital Infection*, **11**: 68–76.

Kirkpatrick JJR, Curtis B, Fitzgerald AM, Naylor IL (1995) A modern translation and interpretation of the treatise on burns of Fabricius Hildanus (1560–1634). *British Journal of Plastic Surgery*, **48**: 460–470.

Kirkpatrick JJR, Naylor IL (1997) Ulcer management in medieval England. *Journal of Wound Care*, **6**: 350–352.

Kranke P, Bennett M, Roeckl-Wiedmann I, Debus S (2004) Hyperbaric oxygen therapy for chronic wounds. *Cochrane Database for Systematic Reviews*, **2**: CD004123.

Lansdown ABG (2004) A review of the use of silver in wound care: facts and fallacies. *British Journal of Nursing*, **13** (suppl): S6-S19.

Leaper DJ, Durani P (2008) Topical antimicrobial therapy of chronic wounds healing by secondary intention using iodine products. *International Wound Journal*, **5**: 361–368.

Lee W, Debastis JC, Lee VK, Lee JH, Fischer K, Edminster K, Park JK, Yoo SS (2009) Multi-layered culture of human skin fibroblasts and keratinocytes through three-dimensional freeform fabrication. *Biomaterials*, **30**: 1587–1595.

Levine JM (1992) Historical notes on pressure ulcers: the cure of Ambroise Paré. *Decubitus*, **5**: 23–26.

Lipsky BA, Hoey C (2009) Topical antimicrobial therapy for treating chronic wounds. *Clinical Practice*, **49**: 1541–1549.

Lineaweaver W, Howard R, Soucy D, McMorris S, Freeman J, Crain C, Robertson J, Rumley T (1985) Topical Antimicrobial Toxicity. *Archives of Surgery*, **120**: 267–270.

Linker RW, Womack N (1969) *Ten Books of Surgery by Ambroise Paré*. Athens: University of Georgia Press.

Löndahl M, Katzman P, Nilsson A, Hammurlund C (2010) Hyperbaric oxygen therapy facilitates healing of chronic foot ulcers in patients with diabetes. *Diabetes Care*, **33**: 1143–1145.

McLure AR, Gordon J (1992) In-vitro evaluation of povidone-iodine and chlorhexidine against methicillin resistant Staphlococcus aureus. *Journal of Hospital Infection*, **21**: 291–299.

Marston WA, Hanft J, Norwood P, Pollack R (2003) The efficacy and safety of Dermagraft in improving the healing of diabetic foot ulcers. *Diabetes Care*, **26**: 1701–1705.

Mayo-Robson AW (1915) Hints on war surgery. *British Journal of Dermatology*, **July 24**: 136.

Meade RH (1968) *An Introduction to the History of General Surgery*. Philadelphia: WB Saunders & Co.

Mengistu Y, Erge W, Bellete B (1999) In vitro susceptibility of gram-negative bacterial isolates to chlorhexidine gluconate. *East African Medical Journal*, **76**: 243–246.

Medical Education Partnership Ltd (2008) Wound infection: principles of best practice. *International Wound Journal*, **5** (suppl 3): 1–11.

Merchant J (1988) Aseptic technique reconsidered. *Care, Science and Practice*, **6**: 74–77.

Michel D, Zach GA (1997) Antiseptic efficacy of disinfecting solutions in suspension test in vitro against methicillin-resistant Staphylococcus aureus, Pseudomonas aeruginosa and Escherichia coli in pressure sore wounds after spinal cord injury. *Dermatology*, **195** (suppl 2): 36–41.

Michaels JA, Campbell B, King B, Palfreyman SJ, Shackley P, Stevenson M (2009) Randomised clinical trial and cost-effective analysis of silver-donating antimicrobial dressings for venous leg ulcers (VULCAN trial). *British Journal of Surgery*, **96**: 1147–1156.

Millward J (1989) Assessment of wound management in a care of the elderly unit. *Care, Science and Practice*, **7**: 47–49.

Morgan D (1995) Myiasis: the rise and fall of maggot therapy. *Journal of Tissue Viability*, **5**: 43–51.

Mouës CM, Vos MC, van den Bemd GJ, Stijen T, Hovius SE (2004) Bacterial load in relation to vacuum-assisted closure: a prospective, randomised trial. *Wound Repair & Regeneration*, **12**: 11–17.

MurrayY (1988) An investigation into the care of wounds in a health authority. *Care Science and Practice*, **6**: 97–102.

Myers JA (1982) Modern plastic surgical dressings. *Health and Social Services Journal*, **92**: 336–337.

Okeniyi JAO, Olubanjo OO, Ogunlesi TA, Oyelami OA (2005) Comparison of healing of incised abscess wounds with honey and EUSOL dressing. *Journal of Alternative and Complementary Medicine*, **11**: 511–513.

Omar AA, Mavor AID, Jones AM, Homer-Vanniasinkam S (2004) Treatment of venous leg ulcers with Dermagraft. *European Journal of Endovascular Surgery*, **27**: 666–672.

O'Toole EA, Goel M, Woodley DT (1996) Hydrogen peroxide inhibits human keratinocyte migration. *Dermatology Surgery*, **22**: 525–529.

Paterson LM (1988) Military surgery: knights, sergeants and Ramon of Avignon's version of Chirugia of Roger of Salerno. In Harper-Bus C, Harvey R eds. *The Ideals and Practice of Medieval Knighthood*. Woodbridge: The Bodell Press.

Phillips PL, Wolcott RD, Fletcher J, Schultz GS (2010) Biofilms made easy. *Wounds International*, **1**: 1–8 (http://woundsinternational.com).

Popp AJ (1995) Crossroads at Salerno: Eldridge Campbell and the writings of Teodorico Borgognoni on wound healing. *Journal of Neurosurgery*, **83**: 174–179.

Redekop WK, McDonnell J, Verboom P, Lovas K, Kalo Z (2003) The cost effectiveness of Apligraf in the treatment of diabetic foot ulcers. *Pharmacoeconomics*, **21**: 1171–1183.

Rees JE (2003) Where have all the bubbles gone? An ode to hydrogen peroxide, the champagne of all wound cleaners. *Accident and Emergency Nursing*, **11**: 82–84.

Reynolds JEF (1982) *Martindale: The Extra Pharmacopoeia*, 28th edn. London: The Pharmaceutical Press.

Rhoads DD, Wolcott RD, Percival SL (2008) Biofilms in wounds: management strategies. *Journal of Wound Care*, **17**: 502–508.

Rode H, Hanslo D, de Wet PM, Millar AJ, Cywes, S. (1989) Efficacy of mupirocin in methicillin-resistant staphylococcu aureus burn wound infection. *Antimicrobial Agents and Chemotherapy*, **33**: 1358–1361.

Russell AD, Hugo WB, Ayliffe GAJ (1982) *Principles and Practice of Disinfection, Preservation and Sterilisation*. London: Blackwell Scientific Publications.

Sander AL, Henrich D, Muth CM, Marzi I, Barker JH, Frank JM (2009) In vivo effect of hyperbaric oxygen on wound angiogenesis and epithelialisation. *Wound Repair & Regeneration*, **17**: 179–184.

Schultz GS, Sibbald RG, Falanga V, Falanga V, Ayello EA, Dowsett C, Harding K, Romanelli M, Stacey MC, Teot L, Vanscheidt W (2003) Wound bed preparation: a systematic approach to wound management. *Wound Repair & Regeneration*, **11**: Suppl): S1–S28.

Sharp A (2009) Beneficial effects of honey dressings in wound management. *Nursing Standard*, **24**: 66–74.

Sherman RA (1997) A new dressing design for use with maggot therapy. *Plastic & Reconstructive Surgery*, **100**: 451–456.

Sinclair RD, Ryan TJ (1993) A great war for antiseptics. *Wound Management*, **4**: 16–18.

Sleigh JW, Linter, S.P.K., (1985) Hazards of hydrogen peroxide. *British Medical Journal*, **291**: 1706.

Tatnall FM, Leigh IM, Gibson JR (1990) Comparative study of antiseptic toxicity on basal keratinocytes, transformed human keratinocytes and fibroblasts. *Skin Pharmacology*, **3**: 157–163.

Thomas S (1990) Eusol revisited. *Dressing Times*, **3**: 3–4.

Thomas S, Jones M, Shutler S, Jones S (1996) Using larvae in modern wound management. *Journal of Wound Care*, **5**: 60–69.

Tredget EE, Shankowsky HA, Groeneveld A, Burrell R (1998) A matched-pair, randomised study evaluating the efficacy and safety of Acticoat™ silver coated dressing for the treatment of burn wounds. *Journal of Burn Care and Rehabilitation*, **19**: 531–537.

Trevelyn J (1997) Spirit of the beehive. *Nursing Times*, **93**: 72–74.

Trilla A, Miro JM (1995) Identifying high risk patients for staphylococcus aureus infections: skin and soft tissue infections. *Journal of Chemotherapy*, **7** (suppl 3): 37–43.

Turner TD (1986) Recent Advances in Wound Management Products. In: Turner TD, Schmidt RJ, Harding KG eds. *Advances in Wound Management*. Chicesther: John Wiley and Sons.

Ubbink DT, Westerbos SJ, Nelson EA, Vermeulen H (2008) A systematic review of topical negative pressure therapy for acute and chronic wounds. *British Journal of Surgery*, **95**: 685–692.

Veves A, Falanga V, Armstrong DG, Sabolinski ML (2001) Graftskin, a human skin equivalent, is effective in the management of noninfected neuropathic diabetic foot ulcers: a prospective multicentre clinical trial. *Diabetes Care*, **24**: 290–295.

Voltaire F (1978) *Zadig and L'Ingenu* (trans Butt J). London: Penguin (first published 1767).

Walsh M, Ford P (1989) *Nursing Rituals, Research and Rational Actions*. Oxford: Heinneman Nursing.

Wasiak J, Cleland H (2007) Topical negative pressure (TNP) for partial thickness burns. *Cochrane Database of Systematic Reviews*, **3**: CD06215.

White RJ, Cutting K, Kingsley A (2006) Topical antimicrobials in the control of wound bioburden. *Ostomy Wound Management*, **52**: 26–58.

Wijesinghe M, Weatherall M, Perrin K, Beasley R (2009) Honey in the treatment of burns: a systematic review and meta-analysis of its efficacy. *New Zealand Medical Journal*, **122**: 47–60.

Wilson JR, Mills JG, Prather ID, Dimitrijevich SD (2005) A toxicity index of skin and wound cleansers used on in-vitro fibroblasts and keratinocytes. *Advances in Skin & Wound Care*, **18**: 373–378.

Wounds UK (2010) *PHMB and its Potential Contribution to Wound Management*. Aberdeen: Wounds UK.

Wright JB, Lam K, Burrell RE (1998) Wound management in an era of increasing bacterial antibiotic resistance: a role for topical silver treatment. *American Journal of Infection Control*, **26**: 572–577.

Zimmerman LM, Veith I (1961) *Great Ideas in the History of Surgery*. Baltimore: Wilkins & Wilkins Co.

5 The Management of Patients with Chronic Wounds

Introduction

Chronic wounds are defined as wounds that have failed to proceed through an orderly and timely reparative process to produce anatomic and functional integrity over a period of 3 months (Mustoe *et al.*, 2006). Despite medical or nursing care they do not heal easily. They are more likely to occur in elderly people or those with multisystem problems.

It cannot be denied that the treatment of chronic wounds is costly. In the UK conservative estimates of the cost to the NHS of chronic wounds puts it at between £2.3 billion and £3.1 billion per year, approximately 3% of total expenditure on health care (Posnett & Franks, 2007). In the USA it has been estimated that chronic wounds affect 5.7 million patients and cost healthcare systems an estimated $20 billion annually (Branski *et al.*, 2009).

Chronic wounds cause much discomfort and pain for the many people who have to suffer them. A multidisciplinary approach is needed for their management and prevention. Nurses can play an important role in the team as they usually have the most contact with the patient. An essential part of this role is communication and cooperation across the disciplines. Healing is not possible for all chronic wounds and in those cases the goal is to assist the patient to achieve the maximum independence and function possible. This chapter will consider the care of patients with pressure ulcers, leg ulcers, diabetic foot ulcers and fungating wounds.

The prevention and management of pressure ulcers

Pressure ulcers are also called pressure sores, bed sores and decubitus ulcers. The most recent definition is that proposed by the National Pressure Ulcer Advisory Panel and the European Pressure Ulcer Advisory Panel in the international pressure ulcer guidelines (NPUAP/EPUAP, 2009):

The Care of Wounds: A Guide for Nurses, Fourth Edition. Carol Dealey.
© 2012 Carol Dealey. Published 2012 by John Wiley & Sons, Ltd.

A pressure ulcer is localized injury to the skin and/or underlying tissue usually over a bony prominence, as a result of pressure, or pressure in combination with shear. A number of contributing or confounding factors are also associated with pressure ulcers; the significance of these factors is yet to be elucidated.

Having been disregarded as merely a nursing problem for many years, there is now a wide acceptance that pressure ulcers have considerable impact on the quality of life of the individual sufferer as well as being a major cost to healthcare services. Two recent qualitative studies have emphasised the fact that pressure ulcers cause pain and distress to patients that can be compounded by the subsequent treatments and the failure of healthcare professionals to acknowledge this (Hopkins *et al.*, 2006; Spilsbury *et al.*, 2007). A systematic review by Gorecki *et al.* (2009) summarised the patients' experience as: severe pain; healthcare professionals ignoring early signs of pressure damage; treatments increasing pain and discomfort; and the social and psychological needs of the patient not being met.

These studies make grim reading for healthcare professionals. Consequently, there is considerable interest in the prevention of pressure ulcers. Prevalence surveys have long been used to determine the size of the pressure ulcer problem in a specific area. They are also used as a quality measure and in benchmarking. This can have financial implications such as the decision by the Center for Medicare and Medicaid Services in the USA that they would no longer pay for the cost of treating hospital or facility-acquired pressure ulcers from October 2008 (van Gilder *et al.*, 2009). In the UK, pressure ulcers have been included in the NHS Commissioning for Quality and Innovation Payment Framework (2008) with local commissioners setting varying targets to reduce the numbers of hospital-acquired pressure ulcers (http://www.institute.nhs.uk/world_class_commissioning/pct_portal/cquin.html).

Whereas on the one hand it is encouraging that pressure ulcer prevention is seen as important at a senior policy level, there is also the problem of a lack of understanding of the complexity in collecting pressure ulcer data and the use of the terms prevalence and incidence as though they are interchangeable.

This problem is well recognised among those working in pressure ulcer prevention and an international group met in 2008 to develop a consensus document providing guidance on measuring prevalence and incidence of pressure ulcers (Medical Education Partnership (MEP), 2009). The document clarifies the differences between prevalence and incidence. Point prevalence 'measures the proportion of a defined set of people who have a pressure ulcer at a particular moment in time'. This includes both those who were admitted to a healthcare facility with a pressure ulcer and those who develop one during their stay. Cumulative incidence or incidence 'indicates the proportion of the population studied that develops new pressure ulcers over a specified time period'. Measuring pressure ulcer incidence is a more accurate measure of the effectiveness of prevention strategies, but it is labour intensive. Prevalence surveys are simpler to undertake, which helps to explain their popularity. Table 5.1 summarises the comparison between prevalence and incidence.

Rather than describe the many prevalence surveys that have been reported over the years, some recent ones are discussed here because of the varying information they provide. Prevalence surveys have regularly been undertaken in North America, Europe, Australia and Japan but Zhao *et al.* (2010) report the first survey undertaken in China. It took place in a 3000-bed teaching hospital in 2009 and the researchers found a point prevalence of 1.8% that reduced to 0.82% when stage 1 pressure ulcers were excluded. This is considerably lower than rates found in North America and Europe, which are around 12% (e.g. van Gilder *et al.*, 2009; James *et al.*, 2010). Zhao *et al.* (2010) suggest that patient acuity is lower in China as patients have a longer average length of stay, but it should also be recognised that effective prevention strategies must play a part.

Table 5.1 **Comparison of prevalence and incidence (reproduced from Medical Education Partnership (2009) with kind permission of MEP Ltd. Full document can be downloaded from www.woundsinternational.com). PU, pressure ulcer**

	Prevalence	Incidence
Description	Measures number of people with *existing* PUs at a given point in time in a specified population	Measures number of people with new PU over a specified period in a specified population
Information provided	Indicates what proportion of the study population had a PU at a given time	Indicates the rate of PU development over a particular time period in a given population
Uses	• Indicates burden of PU • Aids assessment of resource requirements and planning of health services • May collect additional data to aid assessment of compliance with prevention and treatment protocols • Can aid differentiation of community *v.* facility-acquired PUs (with accurate documentation of admission skin assessment)	• Increasingly used as an indicator of quality of care • Study may produce data that prompts a review of factors that contribute to the development of PUs and may therefore suggest prevention strategies • Tracking of comparable incidence rates over time may indicate the effectiveness of prevention measures • May collect additional data to aid assessment of compliance with prevention and treatment protocols
Limitations	Does not provide as direct a measure of quality of care or efficacy of prevention protocols (as does incidence)	May be more time consuming and therefore more expensive than prevalence studies

Sanada *et al.* (2008) reported on the impact of the introduction of a national pressure ulcer prevention strategy in Japan on the prevalence of pressure ulcers, which reduced from 4.26% just before the introduction of the new regulation to 3.64% a year later. Even greater reductions were found by Lahmann *et al.* (2010) in German long-term care facilities where implementation of prevention guidelines reduced pressure ulcer prevalence from 12.5% in 2002 to 5% in 2008. van Gilder *et al.* (2009) found smaller reductions in a large survey undertaken in a variety of healthcare facilities across the USA. The prevalence rate in 2009 was 12.3% in 2009 compared with 13.5% in 2008.

The aetiology of pressure ulcers

Pressure ulcers occur predominantly over the bony prominences, especially the sacrum, ischial tuberosities and heels. Pressure ulcers are caused by a combination of external factors and factors within the patient.

Extrinsic factors

Pressure is the most important factor in pressure ulcer development. Localised, direct pressure causes distortion of the skin and soft tissues that results in tensile and shear stresses near the bony prominence (Takahashi *et al.*, 2010). When the soft tissue of the body is compressed between a bony prominence and a hard surface causing pressures greater than capillary pressure, localised ischaemia occurs. The normal body response to such pressure is to shift position so the pressure is redistributed. When pressure is relieved a red area appears over the bony prominence. This is called reactive hyperaemia and is the result of a temporarily increased blood supply to the area removing waste products and bringing oxygen and nutrients. It is a normal physiological response.

Capillary pressure is generally described as being approximately 32 mmHg, based on the research of Landis (1931). His research was carried out on young, healthy students. He found the average arteriolar pressure was 32 mmHg, but the average pressure in the venules was 12 mmHg. There is also a certain amount of tissue tension that resists deformation. It is not uncommon for interface pressures of around 30–40 mmHg to be seen as 'safe', but this not always correct. Ageing causes a reduction in the numbers of elastic fibres in the tissues, resulting in reduced tissue tension. In situations where the blood pressure is artificially lowered, such as during some types of surgery, capillary pressure is also likely to be lower. In these circumstances, very little pressure is required to cause capillary occlusion. Ek *et al.* (1987) found that a pressure of only 11 mmHg was necessary to cause capillary occlusion in some hemiplegic patients.

If unrelieved pressure persists for a long period of time, tissue necrosis will follow. Prolonged pressure causes distortion of the soft tissues and results in destruction of tissue close to the bone. A cone-shaped ulcer is created, with the widest part of the cone close to the bone and the narrowest on the body surface. Thus, the visible ulcer fails to reveal the true extent of tissue damage.

The role of shear forces in pressure ulcer development is still imperfectly understood, but it is known that shear stresses amplify the effect of pressure in disrupting the local blood supply (Takahashi *et al.*, 2010). Shearing may occur if the patient slides down the bed. The skeleton and tissues nearest to it move, but the skin on the buttocks remains still. One of the main culprits of shearing is the back-rest of the bed which encourages sliding. Chairs that fail to maintain a good posture may also cause shearing.

Friction of itself is not a cause of pressure ulceration, but it contributes to the development of shear forces. Friction occurs when two surfaces rub together. The commonest cause is when the patient is dragged rather than lifted across the bed. It causes the top layers of epithelial cells to be scraped off. Moisture exacerbates the effect of friction. Moisture may be found on a patient's skin as a result of excessive sweating or urinary incontinence.

Intrinsic factors

The human body is frequently subjected to some or all of the extrinsic factors, but does not automatically develop pressure ulcers. The determining factor(s) come from within the patient.

Reduced mobility

This has consistently been shown to be independently predictive of pressure ulcer development in a number of prevalence surveys and epidemiological studies using multivariable analysis (NPUAP/EPUAP, 2009). A typical epidemiological study is that by Lingren *et al.* (2004) who studied a cohort of patients admitted to medical and surgical wards over a 2-year period. They concluded that immobility is a major risk factor for pressure ulcer development among adult hospital patients.

In a seminal study, Exton-Smith and Sherwin (1961) studied the number of movements made by 50 elderly patients during the night. A strong relationship was found between those with reduced movement and the development of pressure ulcers. Reduced movement during sleep may be associated with a variety of drugs such as hypnotics, anxiolytics, antidepressants, opioid analgesics and antihistamines

Another aspect of reduced mobility is that of the patient undergoing major surgery. Operations may last many hours while the patient lies immobile on the operating table. Mobility may be reduced in the immediate post-operative period because of the effects of the anaesthetic, pain, analgesia, infusions or drains. Today very sophisticated surgery is carried out, often on older people and the risks of pressure ulcer development associated with such surgery are consequently increased. Schoonhoven *et al.*

(2002a) observed 208 patients undergoing surgery lasting at least 4 hours and found that 44 (21.2%) developed pressure ulcers within 2 days of surgery. The research team also identified possible risk indicators in these surgical patients and found that the only predictor of pressure ulcer development was length of surgery (Schoonhoven *et al.*, 2002b). A similar study was undertaken by Connor *et al.* (2010) who observed 498 patients undergoing urology surgery of varying types. They found that length of anaesthesia and length of time diastolic blood pressure was below 50 mmHg were statistically significant when loaded together, but concluded this could not be considered clinically relevant without further investigation.

Alterations to intact skin

Alterations to intact skin have also been identified as a risk factor for pressure damage. Fogerty *et al.* (2008) undertook analysis of risk factors for pressure ulcers using the US National In-Patient Sample for 2003, in which a total of 7,977,728 patient discharge diagnoses were available for analysis. They identified deficiency in skin integrity as a significant risk factor. Defloor and Grypdonck (2005) undertook a study of 1772 patients in long-term care facilities over a 4-week period. In one part of the study they undertook logistic regression analysis to determine if any of the items of the Braden or Norton scores were predictors of pressure ulceration development. They found that skin condition and existing pressure ulcers were significant predictors of the development of new pressure ulcers. Nixon *et al.* (2007) undertook a cohort study to identify simple clinical indicators that were independently predictive of >grade 2 pressure ulcer development. They found that non-blanching erythema, especially when associated with localised oedema, induration or pain, to be an independent predictor indicative of advancing pressure damage.

Reduced nutritional status

Reduced nutritional status impairs the elasticity of the skin. Long-term it will lead to anaemia and a reduction of oxygen to the tissues. Poor nutrition has long been considered to be a factor in pressure ulcer development although early research results were inconsistent (Mathus-Vliegen, 2001; Langer *et al.*, 2003). More recent studies have provided more evidence, some looking in general at risk factors and some specifically at malnutrition. Several epidemiological studies identified weight loss, low weight or low body mass index as independent risk factors for pressure ulcer development (e.g. Lingren *et al.*, 2004; Lingren *et al.*, 2005; Nixon *et al.*, 2007). Two large multicentre studies, one in Japan and one in Australia assessed the nutritional status of patients in hospitals, residential care facilities and home care (Lizaka *et al.* 2010; Banks *et al.*, 2010). Both studies found malnutrition to be significantly associated with pressure ulceration. Lizaka *et al.* (2010) also found that malnutrition was strongly associated with more severe pressure ulcers. The factors that may lead to malnutrition are discussed in Chapter 2.

Age

Age has been shown to be a major factor in the development of pressure ulcers as shown by early studies such as David *et al.* (1983) and Nyquist and Hawthorn (1987). More recent epidemiological studies using multivariable methods have found age to be an independent risk factor (Lingren *et al.*, 2004; Lingren *et al.*, 2005; Schoonhoven *et al.*, 2006; Frankel *et al.*, 2007; Fogerty *et al.*, 2008).

As people age, their skin becomes thinner and less elastic. In part, this is because the collagen in the dermis reduces in quantity and quality. Collagen provides a buffer that helps to prevent disruption of the microcirculation (Krouskop, 1983). There may be wasting of the overall body mass, resulting in loose folds of skin. There is also an increased likelihood of chronic illness or disease developing, many of which may also predispose to pressure ulcer development. Once an ulcer occurs it is much harder to heal in an older person than a young one (see Chapter 2).

General health

General health is important as the body can withstand greater external pressure in health than when sick. Bliss (1990) suggested that the acutely ill are particularly vulnerable. Although the reasons for this are not certain, Bliss listed some precipitating factors including pain, low blood pressure, heart failure, the use of sedatives, vasomotor failure, peripheral vasoconstriction due to shock and others. Margolis *et al.* (2003) studied 75,168 older adults on the UK general practitioner research database and identified those with pressure ulcers (1.61%). They found a number of medical conditions that were significantly associated with pressure ulcers: Alzheimer's disease, congestive heart failure, chronic obstructive pulmonary disease, cerebral vascular accident, diabetes mellitus, deep venous thrombosis, hip fracture, hip surgery, limb paralysis, lower limb oedema, malignancy, malnutrition, osteoporosis, Parkinson's disease, rheumatoid arthritis and urinary tract infections. Fogerty *et al.* (2008) found organ or system failure and severe infection to be risk factors for pressure ulcers in their study. Lingren *et al.* (2005) in their study of surgical patients used the American Society of Anesthiologists classification as a pre-operative assessment and found significantly more patients with a score of two or more developed pressure ulcers compared with those with a normal healthy status (a score of one). It is interesting to note that many of these conditions can be found on the list put forward by Bliss (1990) based on her extensive clinical experience.

Neurological or sensory deficit

This may be associated with reduced mobility, such as a patient with paraplegia, but this is not always so. An individual with diabetes may suffer from neuropathy without loss of mobility. Neurological deficit may be associated with strokes, multiple sclerosis, diabetes and spinal cord injury or degeneration. Loss of sensation means the patient is unaware of the need to relieve pressure, even if he is able to do so. Frankel *et al.* (2007) studied risk factors for pressure ulcers in a surgical intensive care unit and found spinal cord injury to be an independent risk factor. Defloor and Grypdonck (2005) considered the individual items in two risk calculators (Braden and Norton) and found sensory perception to be a significant predictor of pressure damage.

Skin moisture

Skin moisture refers to wetness on the skin surface that may be caused by perspiration, incontinence or wound exudate. Both excessive wetness and excessive dryness make the skin less resilient and vulnerable to pressure ulceration. Excessive moisture can weaken the crosslinks between the collagen in the dermis and soften the stratum corneum, resulting in maceration (Clark *et al.*, 2010). In addition, moisture increases the skin's coefficient of friction leading to greater levels of friction and shear stresses (Reger *et al.*, 2010). In contrast, excessively dry skin has lower lipid levels, water content and tensile strength. There is also less flexibility and junctional integrity between the dermis and the epidermis (Clark *et al.*, 2010).

Poor blood supply

Poor blood supply to the periphery lowers the local capillary pressure and causes malnutrition in the tissues. It may be caused by disease, such as heart disease, peripheral vascular disease or diabetes. Frankel *et al.* (2007) found diabetes to be an independent predictor of pressure ulcers in their study of patients in a surgical intensive care unit. Bergstrom *et al.* (1996) found cardiovascular disease to be a significant predictor of pressure ulcer development. Boyle and Green (2001) observed patients in three intensive care units and found that cardiac instability was significantly associated with pressure ulceration. Drugs, such as beta-blockers and inatropic sympathomimetics, may cause peripheral vasoconstriction. These drugs may be used following cardiac surgery when the patient is already suffering from reduced mobility.

Blood flow may also be affected during surgery. Nixon *et al.* (2007) found intra-operative minimum diastolic blood pressure to be an independent predictor of pressure ulceration. Low blood pressure may not just be a problem during surgery, Lingren *et al.* (2004) found it was also a significant risk factor for medical patients. Spittle *et al.* (2001) measured the incidence of pressure ulcers in patients who had undergone lower limb amputations for either ischaemia or neuroischaemia and found an incidence rate of 55% in those who had had major amputations and 20% in minor amputees. They suggest that the presence of peripheral vascular disease may have been a risk factor for these patients. Finally, anaemia has also been identified as a significant risk factor for pressure ulcers in a study of 332 critically ill patients (Theaker *et al.*, 2000).

External factors

Dealey (1997) cited a number of external factors that can exacerbate the factors discussed above. They include:

- inappropriate positioning, which may increase pressure or shear;
- restrictions to movement such as lying for long periods on a trolley;
- lying for long periods in one position on hard surfaces such as the x-ray table;
- poor lifting and handling techniques increase the risk of friction and shear;
- poor hygiene that leaves the skin surface moist from urine, faeces or sweat;
- drugs such as sedatives that make the patient drowsy and less likely to move.

Prevention of pressure ulcers

Although it is a truism, as far as pressure ulcers are concerned, prevention is better than cure. Waterlow (1988) suggested that 95% of all pressure ulcers could be prevented. Although this concept was based on personal opinion, it has been supported by a study undertaken in Japan (Haglsawa & Barbanel, 1999) that observed the outcome of providing preventative care for at-risk patients admitted to an internal medicine ward. The researchers found an incidence rate of 4.4% in the 240 patients they studied. They suggest that this may approach the lowest rate achievable in very ill patients. More recently there has been debate about what constitutes avoidable and unavoidable pressure ulcers. The NPUAP (2010) have provided a definition of an unavoidable pressure ulcer:

> ... the individual developed a pressure ulcer even though the provider had evaluated the individual's clinical condition and pressure ulcer risk factors; defined and implemented interventions that are consistent with individual needs, goals and recognised standards of practice; monitored and evaluated the impact of the interventions; and revised the approaches as appropriate.

In response to the development of evidence-based guidelines, most hospital and primary care trusts use them as a framework from which a local policy may be developed. The most recent pressure ulcer prevention guidelines are those published by the NPUAP and EPUAP and they have been used to inform this section (NPUAP/EPUAP, 2009).

Risk assessment

Risk assessment scales are widely used in risk assessment. Although they are useful tools they should not be used on their own but in conjunction with a comprehensive skin assessment and clinical judgement.

There are a number of risk calculators available. The earliest that was developed was the Norton Score, (Norton *et al.*, 1975). Subsequently other scores have been developed. Probably the most widely used within UK hospitals is the Waterlow score (Waterlow, 1985). This calculator considers a wider range of variables than Norton. The scoring is also reversed so that the higher the score, the higher the risk. The Braden score (Bergstrom *et al.*, 1985) is widely used in the USA and elsewhere and is being increasingly used in the UK. It has been demonstrated to have greater sensitivity and specificity than other scales, but only if used by registered nurses, (Bergstrom *et al.*, 1987).

An interesting systematic review has considered the impact of using a risk calculator on the incidence of pressure ulcers when compared with an unstructured assessment or unaided clinical judgement (Moore & Cowman, 2010). Sadly only one study was considered suitable for inclusion and the reviewers considered it to have a number of methodological problems. To date, therefore, there is very limited high-quality evidence to demonstrate the effectiveness of risk calculators in reducing pressure ulcer incidence. Specific risk factors that require assessment are summarised in Table 5.2.

Table 5.2 **Risk Factors to be included as part of risk assessment (based on NPUAP/EPUAP (2009) with kind permission of the National Pressure Ulcer Advisory Panel © NPUAP)**

Risk factor	Comment
Activity and mobility	Consider anyone who is bed fast and/or chair fast to be at risk
Alterations to intact skin	See skin assessment section
Nutritional indicators	Presence of: anaemia, low haemoglobin or serum albumin, low nutritional intake or weight loss
Factors affecting perfusion and oxygenation	This may include diabetes, cardiovascular instability, poor peripheral perfusion
Skin moisture	Either dry or moist skin
Advanced age	
Potential risk factors:	
• Friction and shear	Subscale Braden Score
• Sensory perception	Subscale Braden Score
• General health status	
• Body temperature	

Risk assessment should not be seen as something that is just part of the initial assessment of a patient, but as something that needs to be repeated on a regular basis, the frequency depending on the condition of the patient. Sudden changes of condition may drastically alter the level of risk of a patient and it is important to undertake a re-assessment of risk. In addition, it must always be remembered that the whole purpose of undertaking a risk assessment is to identify those at risk of developing a pressure ulcer and prevent one occurring. An individualised prevention plan should be instigated without delay. Failure to do so can be classed as negligence.

Skin assessment

Skin assessment is an essential part of assessing patients for their level of risk of pressure ulceration. It is only by actually looking at the skin that we can see signs of incipient pressure damage. Unfortunately skin assessment is often poorly done, skimped or left to untrained staff. It must be acknowledged that early indications of pressure damage are more difficult to identify in patients with darkly pigmented skin and the additional signs of localised heat, oedema or induration may prove useful. There is also some limited evidence that pain over a pressure area is an early indicator of pressure damage, so it is worthwhile identifying any specific areas of pain or discomfort as part of the assessment (Nixon *et al.*, 2006).

It must be acknowledged that the skin status of patients who are terminally ill is especially vulnerable to break down. It may be due to many factors, but Sibbald *et al.* (2010) suggest that impaired tissue perfusion is the most significant and result in dusky erythema or mottled discolouration. Although there has been little research to support practice, there is general agreement on the importance of regular, careful skin assessment in this group of patients.

Nutritional assessment

As has already been discussed, poor nutritional status increases pressure ulcer risk. It is, therefore, important to assess the nutritional status of patients considered to be at risk of pressure ulcer development. Details of nutritional assessment can be found in Chapter 2.

Pressure ulcer prevention strategies

Every patient at risk of pressure ulcer development should have an individualised written plan of care. It is important to document all assessments and the care given. This will enable staff to monitor the effectiveness of the plan and to identify any early signs of tissue damage.

Repositioning

Relief of pressure is the main strategy used in the prevention of pressure ulcers. The commonest method is that of repositioning the patient and traditionally this has been undertaken every 2 hours. Krapfl and Gray (2008) undertook a review of the evidence of the effectiveness of repositioning in reducing pressure ulcer incidence. They found only three studies that met the inclusion criteria: Young (2004), Defloor *et al.* (2005) and Vanderwee *et al.* (2006). The two latter studies looked at different turning regimes on different mattress types and concluded repositioning every 4 hours was equally effective as repositioning every 2 hours when using a visco-elastic mattress. However, Krapfl and Gray noted that in the Vanderwee *et al.* study 34% of patients had spontaneously changed their position in between formal repositioning. It is impossible to determine the impact that this may have had on the outcome of the study. They concluded there is limited evidence to support the use of 4-hourly repositioning in conjunction with a pressure redistributing mattress as opposed to 2-hourly repositioning.

A more recent study examined the association between repositioning and pressure ulcer incidence in a cohort of bed-bound elderly patients with hip fracture (Rich *et al.*, 2011). They did not find that frequent repositioning reduced the incidence of pressure ulcers. However, this was on observational study and the data on repositioning was taken from the nursing charts. There is no certainty that they were accurately maintained.

The Young (2004) study looked the use of the 30° tilt position. This method of positioning patients was developed in a younger-disabled unit (Preston, 1988). The position is achieved by placing pillows in such a manner that the patient's pelvis is tilted at 30°. Once in position, there is no pressure on the sacrum or heels. The interface pressure on the buttock is around 25 mmHg. Patients can be left for increasingly longer periods without turning, again careful observation must be made of all vulnerable areas. Once patients have become accustomed to using the 30° tilt, they may be left for up to 8 hours without turning. This method of positioning is not suitable for all patients as shown by Young (2004) who randomised 46 elderly acutely ill patients to either 30° or 90° lying. She found that many of the patients were unable to maintain the 30° position and questioned the value of the widespread advice to use it. Young also found that 58–61% moved spontaneously in between the times of formal repositioning. Krapfl and Gray (2008) concluded that there is still insufficient evidence to determine the superiority, or otherwise, of the 30° tilt position over either side-lying or the semi-Fowler position.

The use of correct positioning and repositioning techniques, as well as appropriate methods for transferring patients from one surface to another, will reduce both friction and shear forces. Incorrect positions in either bed or chair can cause patients to slide. Regular moving of patients puts nurses at risk of back injury. The European Community has devised regulations on the moving and handling of heavy loads. The directive states that all healthcare institutions must have a policy for manual handling and staff should have regular training on correct methods of moving patients. Hoists, slides and other aids for moving patients should be available. The Royal College of Nursing (2003) produced a code of practice that suggests that manual handling should be eliminated in all but exceptional or life-threatening situations. All nurses have a responsibility to take reasonable care for their own safety and that of patients and colleagues.

When using repositioning as a prevention strategy the following should be considered.

- Frequency of repositioning should be based on the health status of the patient and the treatment plan as well as the support surface in use.
- Consideration should be given the patient's comfort and functional ability.
- Care should be taken to ensure patients are not left lying on medical devices or equipment that could cause localised pressure.
- Regular skin assessment will determine the effectiveness of the repositioning schedule. If there are no signs of improvement or any deterioration over the bony prominences, the prevention plan needs to be reviewed.

Seating – chairs

Most of the research in relation to pressure redistributing equipment has involved mattresses and beds rather than seating, and yet sitting vulnerable patients in armchairs is part of the routine rehabilitation process for many patients (McCafferty et al., 2000). In many instances, hospital armchairs have been purchased without any reference to clinical staff or the varied needs of patients (Collins, 1999; McCafferty et al., 2000). Once ill patients start to sit out of bed, they are perceived to be 'mobile' and so may be left in a chair for long periods of time without being moved and without being able to move much themselves. Gebhardt and Bliss (1994) found prolonged chair sitting increased the incidence of pressure ulcers in orthopaedic patients and it is recommended that the length of time patients sit without pressure relief should be limited (NPUAP/EPUAP, 2009).

Body posture directly affects seating load, so position within a chair is important (van Geffen et al., 2008). Many hospital armchairs have a reclining back of between 15° and 40° that puts the patient in a semi-reclining posture. This may make it more difficult for the patient to stand. Ideally, a chair should have a recline of not more than 10°, enabling the patient to move more freely rather than disabling them (Stockton & Flynn, 2009). Although cushions may be added to chairs to improve pressure relief, the cushion should not make the chair so high that the patient's feet fail to touch the floor. The Tissue Viability Society (TVS) have developed a clinical practice guideline for seating that provides useful information selecting suitable chairs to aid pressure ulcer prevention (Stockton *et al.*, 2009). Conventional seating is not suitable for everyone. Some patients have severe seating problems due to contractures, deformity or infirmity. Specialised seating must be considered for these people.

Support surfaces

Beds, mattresses and overlays

A support surface can be defined as 'a specialised device for pressure redistribution designed for the management of tissue loads, micro-climate and/or other therapeutic functions' (NPUAP, 2007). There is an ever-increasing range of pressure redistributing equipment available for use. They range from overlays to highly sophisticated beds and they can be divided into high-tech and low-tech categories (McInnes *et al.*, 2008). Low-tech devices provide constant low pressure, thus 'spreading the load' and reducing the pressure over bony prominences whereas high-tech devices are dynamic systems with various modes of action. Examples of both high and low-tech devices can be seen in Table 5.3.

High-specification foam mattresses should be used for patients identified as being at risk of pressure ulcer development with an active support surface being selected for those deemed to be at a higher risk (NPUAP/EPUAP, 2009). Consideration should also be given to relieving pressure over the heels that may require the use of an additional heel protection device such as a foam cushion to lift the heels clear of the bed. A small randomised study by Cadue *et al.* (2008) found this device to be effective when compared with no heel intervention. When using this type of device care must be taken to avoid putting pressure on the Achilles

Table 5.3 **Examples of high- and low-tech pressure redistributing devices**

Low tech		High tech	
High spec foam	Overlay	Alternating air	Overlay
	Mattress		Mattress
Gel	Overlay	Low air loss	Overlay
	Mattress		Mattress
Fluid	Overlay		Bed
	Mattress	Air fluidised	Mattress
Fibre	Overlay		Bed
Air	Overlay	Turning beds	Manual controls
	Mattress		Motorised

tendon and to distribute the weight of the leg along the calf (NPUAP/ EPUAP, 2009).

Selection of a suitable support surface should be determined by a number of factors.

- The overall condition of the patient and their ability to mobilise within the bed.
- The overall treatment plan for the patient. A patient who is undergoing rehabilitation may require a different support surface to one who is on bed rest.
- The level of risk of pressure ulcer development.
- The possibility (or otherwise) of the use of regular repositioning. Critically ill patients may be destabilised by repositioning.
- Patient comfort.
- The location of the patient. Not all support surfaces are suitable for home care.

Cushions

Most of the research on cushions has been on those for use in wheelchairs. Wheelchairs have a canvas base, which Rithalia (1989) found exerted pressures in the region of 226 mmHg. It is essential that a cushion should always be used in a wheelchair. For those people who become wheelchair bound because of disability, special assessment should be made to identify the cushion most suited to the specific needs of the patient, taking into consideration the durability of the cushion and the need for it to be replaced (Stockton *et al.*, 2009). Many physiotherapists and occupational therapists have developed specialist skills in assessment. There are many cushions available and information is provided within the TVS guideline about the various types, but there is insufficient evidence to demonstrate whether any cushion outperforms the others and so no specific recommendation can be made (McInnes *et al.*, 2008).

Pressure-relieving devices – other hospital equipment

Vulnerable patients may spend time lying or sitting on very hard surfaces such as operating tables, x-ray tables, trolleys and some types of wheelchair. There is limited research into the use of support surfaces in these areas, other than the use of mattresses on the operating table, but both a visco-elastic pad and an alternating pressure pad have been found to be effective (McInnes *et al.*, 2008).

Skin care

Traditionally, skin care involved rubbing patients' pressure areas at regular intervals. A variety of lotions and potions were used. A review of the literature by Buss *et al.* (1997) considered the effects of massage or rubbing on pressure sore prevention. They concluded that this practice could not be recommended. When the practice of rubbing was discontinued most nurses developed a reluctance to use any type of the cream over the pressure areas. Although this is generally appropriate, there may be exceptions in the case of very dry or very moist skin. Emollients should be considered when caring for patients with very dry skin. This can be in the form of emollients in the bath or an emollient cream. Creams should be applied gently to the affected area. There is limited evidence as to the most effective emollient to use, but one study found a significant difference in pressure ulcer incidence in those randomised to a cream containing hyperoxygenated fatty acids compared with placebo (Bou *et al.*, 2005).

If the skin is moist, the source of the moisture should be identified and dealt with if possible. A systematic review of the prevention and treatment of incontinence-associated dermatitis concluded that frequent cleansing using soap and water for incontinent patients can cause excessive drying of the skin and a skin protectant should be used to protect the skin (Beeckman *et al.*, 2009).

Nutrition

If nutritional assessment identifies a patient as having a reduced nutritional status then an appropriate plan of care must be developed. Chapter 2 discusses this in more detail.

Education and training

There is little point in developing a policy for pressure ulcer prevention if no attempt is made to provide relevant education for healthcare professionals and assistants, patients and carers. A number of authors have described the beneficial outcomes of educational programmes. Sanada *et al.* (2008) reported a significant fall in pressure ulcer prevalence rates in Japan following implementation of government regulated protocols. Orsted *et al.* (2009) described the success of a national quality improvement programme in Canada that reduced incidence rates by up to 71%. Van Gaal *et al.* (2010) undertook a cluster randomised trial to determine the outcome of interactive and tailored education interventions compared with a control and found there was a statistically significant improvement of nurses' knowledge of pressure ulcer prevention.

However, it is not just healthcare professionals who need education. Patients and carers also require information and this should be provided both verbally and in a written format. Information for patients and carers that is written in appropriate language can be obtained from www.nice.org.uk.

Summary

The various aspects of pressure ulcer prevention can be summarised as follows.

- Assessment: identify those at risk, assess and monitor the skin, especially bony prominences.
- Plan appropriate preventative measures.
- Evaluate outcomes by maintaining vigilant skin assessment.
- Monitor all support systems, establishing replacement or maintenance programmes where appropriate.
- Ensure that staff have an adequate knowledge of causes and prevention of pressure ulcers.
- Establish a teaching programme for long term at-risk patients and their carers.
- Monitor outcomes of prevention strategies by measuring the prevalence and incidence of pressure ulcers.

Management of pressure ulcers

If a pressure ulcer occurs, preventative measures should still be continued. The precise cause of the ulcer and the effectiveness of any prevention plan must be evaluated. Any necessary changes must be made, such as using a different support system or increasing proteins and vitamins in the diet. The NPUAP/EPUAP guideline includes assessment, pain assessment, nutritional support, support surfaces, wound management and pressure ulcer management for those receiving palliative care (NPUAP/EPUAP, 2009). Support surfaces and use of devices has been discussed in the previous section, nutrition in Chapter 2 and the principles of wound management can be found in Chapter 3. The rest of the guideline will be used as a framework for this section.

Assessing the pressure ulcer

Determining the severity of a pressure ulcer is an important aspect of developing a treatment plan. It is also required within health service reporting systems, for example, in England and Wales Category 3 and 4 pressure ulcers are classed as indicators in the NHS Outcomes Framework and must be reported (Department of Health, 2010). As part of the international guideline development the NPUAP and EPUAP reviewed the existing methods of grading pressure ulcers and developed a common classification system. Rather than using the terms grading or staging that both imply a progression from one through to four, it was decided to use a more non-hierarchical word, category instead (NPUAP/EPUAP, 2009). The new classification system is detailed below.

Category I: non-blanchable erythema
Intact skin with non-blanchable redness of a localised area usually over a bony prominence. Darkly pigmented skin may not have visible blanching; its colour may differ from the surrounding area. The area may be painful, firm, soft, warmer or cooler as compared with adjacent tissue. Category I may be difficult to detect in individuals with dark skin tones. May indicate 'at-risk' individuals.

Category II: partial thickness
Partial thickness loss of dermis presenting as a shallow open ulcer with a red-pink wound bed, without slough. May also present as an intact or open/ruptured serum-filled or sero-sanginous filled blister. Presents as a shiny or dry shallow ulcer without slough or bruising (bruising indicates deep tissue injury). This category should not be used to describe skin tears, tape burns, incontinence associated dermatitis, maceration or excoriation.

Category III: full-thickness skin loss
Full-thickness tissue loss. Subcutaneous fat may be visible but bone, tendon or muscle is *not* exposed. Slough may be present but does not obscure the depth of tissue loss. *May* include undermining and tunnelling. The depth of a Category III pressure ulcer varies by anatomical location. The bridge of the nose, ear, occiput and malleolus do not have (adipose) subcutaneous tissue and Category III ulcers can be shallow. In contrast, areas of significant adiposity can develop extremely deep Category III pressure ulcers. Bone/tendon is not visible or directly palpable.

Category IV: full-thickness tissue loss
Full-thickness tissue loss with exposed bone, tendon or muscle. Slough or eschar may be present. Often includes undermining and tunnelling. The depth of a Category IV pressure ulcer varies by anatomical location. The bridge of the nose, ear, occiput and malleolus do not have (adipose) subcutaneous tissue and these ulcers can be shallow. Category IV ulcers can extend into muscle and/or supporting structures (e.g., fascia, tendon or joint capsule) making osteomyelitis or osteitis likely to occur. Exposed bone/muscle is visible or directly palpable.

Additional categories
Unstageable/unclassified: full-thickness skin or tissue loss – depth unknown: full-thickness tissue loss in which actual depth of the ulcer is completely obscured by slough (yellow, tan, gray, green or brown) and/or eschar (tan, brown or black) in the wound bed. Until enough slough and/or eschar are removed to expose the base of the wound, the true depth cannot be determined; but it will be either a Category III or IV. Stable (dry, adherent, intact without erythema or fluctuance) eschar on the heels serves as 'the body's natural (biological) cover' and should not be removed.

Suspected deep tissue injury – depth unknown: purple or maroon localised area of discoloured intact skin or blood-filled blister due to damage of underlying soft tissue from pressure and/or *shear*. The area may be preceded by tissue that is painful, firm, mushy, boggy, warmer or cooler as compared with adjacent tissue. Deep tissue injury may be difficult to detect in individuals with dark skin tones. Evolution may include a thin blister over a dark wound bed. The wound may further evolve and become covered by thin eschar. Evolution may be rapid exposing additional layers of tissue even with optimal treatment.

Figure 5.1 shows examples of each of these categories of pressure ulcer.

Difficulties with classifying ulcers

There are a number of issues that need to be considered when utilising any classification system: accurate identification of category I ulcers, incontinence-associated dermatitis and reverse grading.

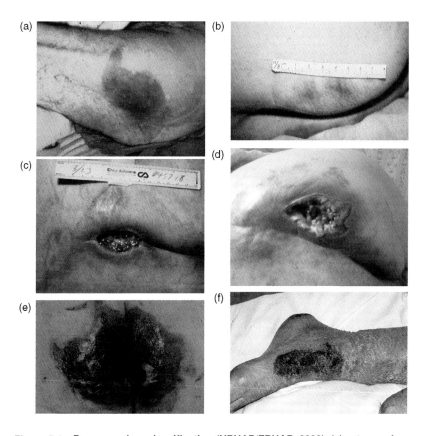

Figure 5.1   **Pressure ulcer classification (NPUAP/EPUAP, 2009). (a) category I; (b) category II; (c) category III; (d) category IV; (e) deep tissue injury; (f) unstageable**

Category I pressure ulcers are often found to account for approximately 50% of all ulcers in prevalence surveys (e.g. van Gilder *et al.*, 2008; Zhao *et al.*, 2010). However, there are problems with both over- and under-reporting. Over-reporting may occur if nurses fail to differentiate between blanching and non-blanching erythema. Alternatively, under-reporting may occur because of the difficulties in identifying erythema on dark skin (Scanlon & Stubbs, 2004; van Gilder *et al.*, 2008). Attempts have been made to provide additional descriptors to the definition as can be seen above. However, there is a need to undertake further research to identify a truly accurate method of assessment that overcomes skin colour.

Incontinence-Associated Dermatitis (IAD) is sometimes mistaken for pressure ulcers (Defloor & Schoonhoven, 2004; Defloor *et al.*, 2006). Incontinence can cause erythema, excoriation and maceration of the skin and thus an incontinence lesion may have a similar appearance to a category II or III pressure ulcer. Care should be taken to determine the precise position of any ulcerated skin in incontinent patients. If is not over a bony prominence, it is more likely to be as a result of incontinence rather than pressure.

Reverse grading or staging is the practice of describing a healing pressure ulcer as moving from a category IV, through category III and then to category II as a pressure ulcer cavity heals and becomes shallower. The American NPUAP debated this topic and produced a position statement that can be found at www.npuap.org, this states that as pressure ulcers heal they fill with granulation tissue that is not the same as the tissue that it replaces, therefore reverse staging should not be used. A category IV pressure ulcer should therefore be described as a healing category IV ulcer.

The location of pressure ulcers

Some bony prominences are more prone to pressure ulcers than others. The sacrum, heels and buttocks are the most commonly reported locations (e.g. Clark *et al.*, 2003; van Gilder *et al.*, 2008; Zhao *et al.*, 2010). There are also reports of medical device-related pressure damage. Van Gilder *et al.* (2009) found 9% of all pressure ulcers were related to devices in their study of 17,911 pressure ulcers. Most commonly they were located on the ear.

There are some specific aspects of care that need to be considered.

- *Sacrum*: dressings must be chosen with care, as many tend to ruckle up as the patient moves. Chair sitting must be strictly regulated as to type of chair and length of time seated in it.
- *Buttocks*: as for sacrum.
- *Heels*: ideally dressings must not be too bulky as this may impede mobility. Dressings may need to be 'tailored' in order to fit correctly

around the heel. If footwear is being worn, care must be taken to ensure that it is not too tight, or this will exert pressure on foot. Ensure there is adequate pressure relief when in bed.

- *Trochanters*: some dressings may ruckle up, select carefully.
- *Elbows*: these pressure ulcers are usually caused by friction from moving about the bed. Consider ways of reducing friction – use of a monkey pole, use of pads or semi-permeable film dressings.
- *Trunk*: ulcers here are uncommon, try and identify source of pressure and remove or modify it.

Wound bed

Wound bed management has been discussed in detail in Chapter 3. The same principles can be applied to pressure ulcers. A pressure ulcer should be assessed for its appearance as well as its category. Accurate assessment is necessary in order to select a suitable wound management product.

Pain assessment

Patients with pressure ulcers experience both ulcer-related pain and treatment-related pain (Hopkins *et al.*, 2006; Spilsbury *et al.*, 2007). Patients should be assessed for pain and a management plan developed. This has been discussed in Chapters 2, 3 and 4.

Selection of wound management products

A variety of wound management products can be used when treating pressure ulcers. The range of wound management products that are available are discussed in Chapter 4. The evidence for each dressing type was reviewed for the international pressure ulcer guidelines and guidance given for the use of each of the main dressing types (NPUAP/ EPUAP, 2009).

A literature review by Lohi *et al.* (2010) considered studies from 2000 to 2008 and concluded that hydrocolloids are the most widely used treatment for pressure ulcers. Heyneman *et al.* (2008) undertook a systematic review of the use of hydrocolloid dressings to treat pressure ulcers and found they were significantly more effective than saline-soaked gauze. However, when compared with other modern products such as alginates, foams, topical enzymes and a biosynthetic dressing, hydrocolloids were significantly less effective.

A cost-effectiveness study was undertaken to compare the cost of using a thin foam dressing with saline-soaked gauze to treat category II pressure ulcers (Payne *et al.*, 2009). A total of 36 patients were randomised to either treatment and monitored for 4 weeks. The cost of using the foam dressing were significantly lower than using gauze and there were also more ulcer-free days in the foam group. The study was not powered to detect a difference in healing rates.

The use of plastic surgery

The healing time of a large cavity pressure ulcer can be considerably reduced by plastic surgery. However, it is not appropriate for all patients. Their condition may be too poor or the ulcer may be healing rapidly. Sorensen *et al.* (2004) suggest that only a small proportion of patients are suitable candidates, generally, those with spinal cord injury deep category III or IV ulcers. Srivastava *et al.* (2009) discussed the importance of treating the patient as a whole and incorporating the surgery into the rehabilitation process. The first stage of reconstruction is debridement followed by either simple closure or use of a flap. If a wound is heavily colonised, it is best to undertake reconstruction in two separate stages, so that there is an opportunity to reduce the bacterial count (Sorensen *et al.*, 2004). Singh *et al.* (2010) looked at a number of additional outcomes besides healing following surgery for pressure ulcers in 30 spinal cord injured patients. They found that there was a general improvement in quality of life and a significant improvement in haemoglobin, serum albumin and total serum proteins levels at 6 months post surgery.

The major problem with reconstruction surgery is the high rate of recurrence. Tavakoli *et al.* (1999) found a recurrence rate of 62% when monitoring outcomes over an 8-year period. However, Kierney *et al.* (1998) found that such rates could be reduced by working collaboratively with colleagues in the department of physical medicine and rehabilitation. In a longitudinal study of 158 patients they found a recurrence rate of 25%. They considered their success was related to improved patient selection combined with a protocol for rehabilitation following surgical repair. Keys *et al.* (2010) reviewed 135 spinal cord injured patients undergoing reconstructive surgery and used multivariable analysis to identify predictors of flap failure. They found that early recurrence was associated with poor nutrition and poorly controlled diabetes. Late recurrence was associated with young age (under 45 years), ischial wound location and previous operative failure on the same site. Addressing these issues could assist in improving outcomes following surgery.

Palliative care

Patients at the end of life are very vulnerable to pressure damage and although healing may occur, it may not be a realistic goal for all patients (NPUAP/EPUAP, 2009). The main goals are patient comfort and limiting the impact of the pressure ulcers in accordance with the patient's wishes (Bates-Jenson *et al.*, 2004). The international pressure ulcer guidelines provide extensive guidance on the management and care of this group of patients (NPUAP/EPUAP, 2009).

Summary

The various aspects of pressure ulcer management can be summarised as follows:

- identify the causative factors and remove/address where possible;
- assess the pressure ulcer for severity, location and wound bed appearance;
- assess for other aspects such as nutritional status and pain;
- determine the goals of care for the patient;
- select a suitable support system;
- develop a wound management plan that includes wound management, nutritional support and pain management;
- monitor the outcomes and review care if necessary.

The management of leg ulcers

Leg ulcers are a very common type of chronic wound that has been recognised for many years. Modern developments in wound management have revitalised those caring for patients with leg ulcers.

The epidemiology of leg ulcers

Undertaking prevalence surveys of leg ulcers is more complex than pressure ulcers. The majority of people with leg ulcers are in the community and it is suggested that possibly as many of 44% of them manage their ulcers themselves (Nelzen *et al.*, 1996b). This figure may be even higher in those who are working and do not want to take time off work to attend clinics (Nelzen *et al.*, 1996a). Therefore studies that do not include self-reporting may only be reflecting the healthcare burden rather than the burden of the disease (Firth *et al.*, 2010). However, including self-reporting requires multiple strategies to collect valid data and is more time-consuming and costly to undertake (Firth *et al.*, 2010).

It seems reasonable to question if the perceived wisdom regarding the epidemiology of leg ulcers may be an underestimation, although some prevalence studies have used self-reporting. Two reviews of leg ulcer surveys were published in 2003 (Briggs & Closs, 2003; Graham *et al.*, 2003). They did not review exactly the same surveys as their search time-frames were slightly different, but they did draw similar conclusions. Using the most reliable estimates from studies undertaken in Europe, Australia and USA, Briggs and Closs (2003) concluded that the prevalence of open ulcers is around 0.11–0.18% whereas Graham *et al.* (2003) found it to be

0.12–1.1%. Briggs and Closs (2003) also found that those suffering from recurrent leg ulceration were about 1–2% of the population. These figures should not be extrapolated to other parts of the world where the prevalence rates may be entirely different.

The figures from prevalence surveys such as those quoted above should not be seen as static. Prevalence rates may change over time because of the impact of improved care and changes in disease burden. Forssgren *et al.* (2008) replicated a prevalence survey originally undertaken in 1988 with the second survey being conducted in 2002. The surveys were conducted in one county in Sweden where there is a large elderly population. They found a point prevalence of 2.4/1000 population in 2002 compared with a point prevalence of 3.1/1000 in 1988. This represents a 23% reduction in the prevalence of leg ulcers. There was also a change in leg ulcer aetiology as the numbers of venous and arterial ulcers had decreased and the numbers of diabetic ulcers and those caused by multiple factors had increased (Forssgren *et al.*, 2008). The authors concluded that these changes reflected improved organisation of care for leg ulcer patients, lower recurrence rates following increased use of venous surgery and an increase in the numbers of people with diabetes.

One of the problematic features of leg ulcers is the length of time they can take to heal and the frequency of recurrence. Purwins *et al.* (2010) studied 218 people with chronic leg ulcers and found that they had suffered from leg ulcers for a mean of 14 years (range 0–61 years; median 6 years).

The cost of leg ulcers

As has already been shown, leg ulcers can be a longstanding and recurrent problem. Inevitably, they are also very expensive. The majority are cared for in the community and so require home visits or to be taken to clinics, the worst cases may be admitted to hospital. Friedberg *et al.* (2002) undertook a survey over 4 weeks of home care nurses visiting leg ulcer patients in a large urban setting in Canada. She found that the mean travel and visit times cost in Candian dollars was $80.62 and the mean supply costs were $21.06. A total of 2270 visits were made in the study period and the annual costs were estimated to be around $1.3 million. Tennvall *et al.* (2004) calculated the cost of treating venous ulcers in Sweden based on existing epidemiological data. They found the annual cost to be €73 million. A study undertaken in 23 specialist leg ulcer centres in Germany looked at both direct and indirect costs (Purwins *et al.*, 2010). Direct costs were those relating to ulcer treatment and the indirect costs related to loss of earnings, inability to work, early retirement and so on. The mean total annual cost per patient was €9569, most of which was direct costs (€8658.10) with indirect costs amounting to €911.20.

Several centres have established community leg ulcer clinics and costed the outcomes. Patton (2009) undertook a review of the topic and concluded that although there were greater costs associated with leg ulcer clinics, this was mitigated by faster healing times. Overall, this made the clinics cost-effective, but there could be further gains if more education was provided for all home care nurses, not just those working in the leg ulcer clinics.

None of the studies quoted above consider the cost to the patient. Such costs are impossible to quantify. Several researchers have investigated the cost to the patient. Persoon *et al.* (2004) undertook a review of the literature to determine the impact of leg ulceration on daily life. They included 37 studies, both qualitative and quantitative methodologies. The common problem identified in all studies is pain and a number also identified disturbed sleep associated with pain, for example, Hofman *et al.* (1997) interviewed 94 patients with venous ulcers and found that 64% had severe pain, 38.3% had continuous pain and 63.8% were woken by pain. Another problem identified by the reviewers is impaired mobility. The reviewers conclude that leg ulceration has a major impact on the life of the sufferer. A more recent study (Jones *et al.*, 2008) used the Hospital Anxiety and Depression Scale for 196 patients with leg ulcers and found 27% ($n = 52$) were depressed and 26% ($n = 50$) were anxious. Twenty of these patients were then interviewed using a phenomenological approach. Analysis of the interviews showed that the patients experienced feelings of shame, disgust and self-loathing due to the exudate and odour from their ulcer. They were afraid that others would notice the odour and so limited their social activities. The patients also described the problems of coping with leakage on the outside of their bandages, particularly a problem when the bandages were only changed weekly.

Leg ulcer aetiology

There are a variety of causes of leg ulcers. The commonest are venous disease and arterial disease. O'Brien *et al.* (2000) surveyed a health district in Ireland and found 81% of ulcers were venous in origin and 16.3% were due to arterial disease. Forssgren *et al.* (2008) found that although the prevalence of venous ulcers had reduced by 46% and arterial ulcers by 23% in their 2002 survey, they were still the most common cause of leg ulcers. Around 9% of patients with leg ulcers have rheumatoid arthritis and although they could have ulcers associated with their disease, they could also have venous or arterial ulcers (Scottish Intercollegiate Guideline Network, 2010). Increasingly, more complex aetiologies are being identified, perhaps because of increasing age and also improved management of the straightforward cases.

Venous ulceration

Aetiology

Chronic venous insufficiency is the main cause of venous leg ulcers. Initially, thrombosis or varicosity causes damage to the valves in the veins of the leg. The deep vein is surrounded by muscle. When the leg is exercised, the calf muscle contracts and squeezes the veins, encouraging the flow of blood along the vein. This is often referred to as the calf muscle pump.

Normally blood flows from the superficial veins to the deep veins via a series of perforator vessels. The valves in the vessels ensure that blood moves from the capillary bed towards the heart. If some of the valves become damaged then blood can flow in either direction. The backflow of blood towards the capillary bed leads to venous hypertension. As a result, the capillaries become distorted and more permeable. Larger molecules than normal are able to escape into the extravascular space, for example fibrinogen and red blood cells. The haemoglobin is first released from the red blood cells and then broken down causing eczema and a brown staining in the gaiter area. Ultimately there is fibrosis of the underlying tissues giving the leg a 'woody' feeling. This condition is called lipodermatosclerosis. The slightest trauma to the leg and an ulcer will develop. Common examples of trauma are knocking the leg on the corner of a piece of furniture or a fall, injuring the lower leg.

The lymphatic system may also be affected. The lymphatics are responsible for removing protein, fat, cells and excess fluid from the tissues. Ryan (1987) has described how the superficial lymphatics in the dermis disappear. This results in waste products accumulating in the tissues, which can cause fibrosis and further oedema.

Management

Assessment – the patient
Full assessment of the patient is essential as many factors can delay the healing of chronic wounds, (see Chapter 2). A medical assessment may be necessary to ensure accurate diagnosis. The leg ulcer guidelines developed by the Scottish Intercollegiate Guideline Network (SIGN) suggest a number of factors that may be specifically indicative of venous ulceration and those that are indicative of other aetiologies (SIGN, 2010). They can be seen in Table 5.4. Other factors that may need to be particularly considered include nutritional status, mobility, sleeping, pain, psychological effects of leg ulceration and the patient's understanding of the disease process.

Assessment – the leg
A comprehensive assessment of the affected leg must be made, as it is important to rule out arterial disease. The treatments for these two types of ulcer are not compatible. First look at the legs. The characteristic staining of lipodermatosclerosis is usually clearly seen in the gaiter area. Ankle flare may also be present. This is distension of the network of small veins situated just below the medial malleolus. Oedema may be present, but can also be found in arterial ulceration. Theoretically, the leg and foot should feel warm

Table 5.4   **Factors to include in assessment of patients with leg ulceration**

Factors indicative of venous ulceration	Factors indicative of non-venous ulceration
Family history	Family history of non-venous ulcers
Varicose veins	Heart disease, stroke, TIA
Proven DVT in affected leg	Diabetes mellitus
Phlebitis in affected leg	Ischaemic rest pain
Pregnancy	Hypertension
Suspected DVT	Bypass surgery
Surgery/fractures to the leg	Rheumatoid arthritis
Leg infection	Peripheral vascular disease/intermittent claudication

DVT, deep vein thrombosis; TIA, transient ischaemic attack.

to touch, but if the weather is cold this may not be the case. The skin surrounding the ulcer may be fragile and eczematous.

Typically, venous ulcers are found on or near the medial malleolus. They tend to be shallow and develop slowly over a period of time. It should also be noted that pain will be increased if there is any infection in the ulcer. The ulcer appearance should be assessed as in Chapter 3. Many venous ulcers have a heavy exudate. Figure 5.2 shows a typical venous ulcer with staining in the gaiter area.

Differential diagnosis between venous and arterial ulcers can be achieved by assessing the blood supply to the leg, ideally by means of Doppler ultrasound. This procedure should be undertaken by healthcare

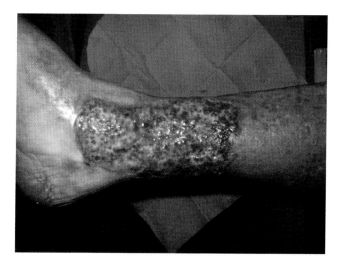

Figure 5.2   **A venous ulcer**

professionals who have received training so to do. The Doppler is used to compare the blood pressure in the lower leg with the brachial pressure. It is usually presented in the form of a ratio, the ankle brachial pressure index (ABPI), which is calculated by the following formula:

$$\frac{\text{ankle systolic pressure}}{\text{brachial systolic pressure}} = \text{ankle brachial pressure index}$$

An ABPI of 0.9 or above indicates a normal arterial supply to the leg. If it is below 0.9 then some ischaemia is present. Compression therapy should not be used if the ABPI is below 0.8. Patients with diabetes may have calcified blood vessels, leading to a falsely high reading. Clinical decisions should not be made based on ABPI results over 1.5 (SIGN, 2010). If there is any doubt about the presence of arterial disease, further medical opinion should be sought.

Assessment – the ulcer
The ulcer should be assessed as discussed in Chapter 3.

Assessment – the surrounding skin
Although assessment of the surrounding skin has been discussed in Chapter 3, there are some very specific issues for patients with leg ulcers. Varicose eczema is commonly found in these patients, causing erythema, weeping and scaling and is sometimes mistaken for infection (SIGN, 2010). Another problem due to the longevity of many ulcers is allergic contact dermatitis. The SIGN guideline recommends that patients with either varicose eczema or dermatitis should be patch tested using a leg ulcer series. Cameron (1998) reviewed the problems of allergic contact dermatitis or contact sensitivity. Substances which have been found to cause sensitivities include lanolin, neomycin, framycetin, emulsifiers such as cetyl alcohol, latex, parabens and colophony. Machet *et al.* (2004) reviewed changes in sensitivities reported in France since 1990 and found an 8.5% increase in sensitivity rates. There was a slight decrease in sensitivity to lanolin and a marked increase in sensitivity to balsam of Peru.

Determining the relevant allergens is important when planning an appropriate management plan as it may be the ingredients of specific dressings or bandages that are the sensitiser.

Planning
There are three aspects to the management of venous ulcers: the use of appropriate wound management products, skin care and improving the drainage of the leg. Any one of these alone will not be truly effective without the others.

Wound Management: management of the ulcer depends on assessment 4 and the factors previously discussed. Selection of suitable dressings is discussed in Chapter 4. There have been a number of clinical trials looking at the use of modern products for managing leg ulcers, many of which have been of a small size or inconclusive. A recent systematic review (Palfreyman *et al.*, 2010) found 23 studies of hydrocolloid dressings compared with much fewer studies of other dressings, for example 6 studies of foam dressings. The reviewers concluded that the evidence showed no difference in the effectiveness of hydrocolloids or simple non-adherent dressings in respect of healing. There was insufficient evidence to reach a conclusion about the other dressing types.

Alginates, foams and hydrogels have also been widely used, especially to manage exudate or slough. Dumville *et al.* (2009) found that larval therapy significantly reduced the time to debridement compared with a hydrogel in a study of 267 patients with a variety of venous, arterial and mixed aetiology ulcers. Marston and Vowden (2003) suggest that dressing selection should be based on the status of the ulcer and surrounding skin. It should be remembered that while the ulcer may be new to the nurse, the patient could have lived with it for some time. There may be a credibility gap as the patient starts yet another course of treatment that will definitely resolve the problem.

Skin grafts are used in some centres to promote faster healing. Either mesh grafts or pinch grafts may be used, but the former requires hospital admission. Grafting should be used in conjunction with compression therapy. A Cochrane review assessed the benefits of skin grafts, including tissue culture and bilayer artificial skin (Jones & Nelson, 2007). They concluded that bilayer artificial skin and compression healed more ulcers than a simple dressing and compression. Further research is needed to determine the usefulness of other forms of skin grafts. Margolis *et al.* (2000) suggested using a simple prognostic model to identify those patients who would not heal with a simple dressing plus compression bandaging within 24 weeks. Those identified could then be considered for more sophisticated treatment, such as artificial skin.

Skin care: management of the ulcer involves cleansing and a suitable topical application. Consideration must be given to the presence of eczema, scaling on the legs around the ulcer, any allergies to treatment and wound infection. Footbaths are very useful as they allow the patient the opportunity to give the affected leg a good soak. Plain tap water is suitable for most patients. Attention needs to be paid to the adequate cleansing of the footbath after use in order to prevent cross-infection. Bland emollients such as a 50/50 mixture of soft white paraffin and liquid paraffin should be applied following cleansing of the leg. This can be massaged gently into the skin, helping to lift the skin scales that rapidly build up on the leg. Emollients and topical steroids may be used to treat eczema and care must be taken to avoid any irritants that may aggravate the eczema (SIGN, 2010).

Drainage of the legs: this can be improved in several ways: exercise, compression and elevation. The use of exercise stimulates the calf muscle pump, promoting drainage. Two studies have shown improvement in calf muscle function by using simple exercises such as heel raises (Kan & Delis, 2001; Jull *et al.*, 2009). Neither study was long enough or large enough to see if this would translate into ulcer healing, but such an outcome would seem logical. Obviously exercise should be tailored to the abilities of the patient. Regular encouragement will be needed to ensure patients persist with their exercises.

Compression works with exercise to aid drainage from the superficial veins. It should be graduated so that there is a higher pressure at the ankle than at the calf. It can be achieved by the use of either bandages or stockings. Bandages are probably easiest to use in the early stages when the dressings may be rather bulky. Some remain *in situ* day and night whereas others may be removed at night. When re-applying bandages it is best done before rising when the leg has the least amount of oedema.

The World Union of Wound Healing Societies (WUWHS) has produced a consensus statement on the use of compression that provides useful guidance on the terminology used to describe compression bandages (WUWHS, 2008). They suggest that as all bandages overlap when they are applied a single layer bandage does not exist. The expert working group preparing the document propose using the term multicomponent system to describe the combination of padding and bandages being used. They also suggest that ankle circumference and the target sub-bandage pressure or level of bandage stiffness should be recorded (WUWHS, 2008).

The level of compression needed for venous ulceration is around 40 mmHg, (Stemmer, 1969). Therefore, the high compression bandages are generally suitable. However, these pressures are dependent on the size of the limb. A large limb, swollen with oedema, would require a higher compression bandage than a thinner limb in order to achieve an adequate level of compression. There is also a need to ensure protection over bony prominences as there is the potential risk of pressure damage, especially if the bandage is poorly applied.

A systematic review of clinical trials of compression bandaging found venous ulcers heal more rapidly with compression than with no compression (O'Meara *et al.*, 2009). The same review also found that multicomponent systems were more effective than single systems and systems including an elastic bandage layer seem to be more effective than those containing mainly inelastic components.

Unfortunately, not all patients can tolerate high compression bandage systems and a pragmatic approach to the problem may be necessary. The WUWHS (2008) have proposed some practical solutions to address the challenges associated with the use of compression bandages and the need to meet patients' individual requirements.

Compression stockings may be used as an alternative to bandages. They have the advantage that they are less bulky than bandages, allowing patients to wear more usual shoes. They also require less skill to apply than bandages, which may be an advantage. Some manufacturers also produce compression socks for men that look like ordinary socks. The British Standards Institute has specified three classes of stockings that are available on prescription. The three classes provide different ranges of compression at the ankle:

- Class I Has pressures of 14–18 mmHg
- Class II has pressures of 18–24 mmHg
- Class III has pressures of 25–35 mmHg

It is very important that the patient should be correctly fitted for a stocking. The WUWHS (2008) suggest that a two-component system is safer and easier to use than a single stocking. The first stocking (e.g. Class I) holds the dressing in place and the second stocking (e.g. Class II) can be removed at night. The major disadvantage of stockings is they are not suitable if the ulcer is exuding heavily and needs a bulky dressing. A systematic review by Amsler *et al.* (2009) of eight studies found that a significantly greater number of ulcers healing with stockings and the average time to healing was shorter by 3 weeks.

Another method of applying compression that can be used, particularly if oedema is present, is pneumatic compression. It may be applied once or twice a day for periods of up to an hour. Initially the time should be shorter and gradually increased. Although this may be a useful form of treatment, it is difficult in the community where there is limited access to such equipment. The use of pneumatic compression should be seen as an addition to the treatment regime rather than an alternative. A Cochrane review found limited evidence of benefits of pneumatic compression and concluded that it may increase healing compared with no compression, but further research is required to determine if it increases healing rates (Nelson *et al.*, 2008).

Elevation of the legs allows gravity to aid venous return. However, many people tend to place their feet on a low stool, which is of no benefit whatsoever. To be effective the feet should be higher than the heart. If there is an acute exacerbation of the ulcer with oedema and heavy exudate, it may be worthwhile to admit the patient to hospital so that he/she may have a short period of bed rest. Bed rest with elevation of the foot of the bed can significantly reduce oedema and improve venous return. It should not be considered as a long-term measure because the ulcer will merely break down again once the patient is up and about. It may also seriously affect the mobility of older patients. A more practical method is to raise the foot of the bed at home so that the legs are elevated at night-time. This may be achieved by the use of bricks or blocks of wood.

It is well recognised that a considerable number of patients do not comply with their treatment regime, particularly with their compression therapy. Two reviews have considered the literature in relation to this lack of concordance from both the patient and healthcare perspective (Moffatt *et al.*, 2009; van Hecke *et al.*, 2009). A wide range of factors were identified that included: compression being bulky, causing discomfort or pain; conflicting advice from healthcare professionals; lack of understanding of condition or treatment; lack of motivation by patient. Inevitably this has a negative impact on healing that in itself may increase non-concordance. Van Hecke *et al.* (2009) suggest that compliance with treatment is a shared responsibility involving both patients and healthcare professionals and it is important that nurses have a clear understanding of the problems faced by patients in order to develop a mutually agreed treatment plan.

Additional treatments: pentoxifylline is a drug that improves blood flow through peripheral blood vessels and therefore helps with blood circulation in the arms and legs (e.g. intermittent claudication), and the brain. It is sometimes used to treat venous leg ulcers either with or without compression. A systematic review by Jull *et al.* (2007) found that pentoxifylline is effective when treating venous ulcers with compression and may be effective for those not receiving compression.

Evaluation

Regular assessment of the ulcer may be done by the use of tracings or photographs. They are essential to monitor the progress of the ulcer. Healing of venous leg ulcers is not quick and it is generally accepted that venous ulcers can take a minimum of 3 months to heal and that the longer an ulcer is open, the longer it will take to heal. However, if there appears to be no progress over a period of 2–3 months the ulcer should be re-assessed and a vascular opinion may be necessary. Neequaye *et al.* (2009) studied a group of 122 non-healing ulcers and found that a history of deep vein thrombosis (DVT) and widespread deep reflux were associated with ulcers open for more than a year.

Prevention of recurrence

Once an ulcer is healed there is still the risk of recurrence with studies showing 60–70% recurrence rates (Finlayson *et al.*, 2009). A study of 122 patients with healed leg ulcers found that many of the participants (68%) had had recurrence of ulceration, particularly in the first 3 months (36%) (Finlayson *et al.*, 2009). The research team also found that those who elevated their legs for an hour per day were 25-times less likely to have an occurrence than those who did not. In addition, they also found that for every day or week patients wore either Class II or III compression stockings the ulcers were half as likely to recur. This finding is supported by a systematic review of the use of compression hosiery for preventing ulcer recurrence (Nelson *et al.*, 2010). The reviewers noted that not wearing compression was strongly associated with leg ulcer recurrence, although this is circumstantial evidence as this condition was not being tested in trials. In a further paper Finlayson *et al.* (2010) describe using multivariable analysis to determine factors that would influence wearing of compression hosiery. They found that self-efficacy, knowledge and depression were significant factors; those unable to provide self-care, lacking knowledge of their condition or with depression were more likely to have a recurrence.

Surgery may be used to correct superficial venous reflux once the ulcer is healed. The ESCHAR study randomised 500 patients with open or recently healed ulcers to either compression or compression with surgery and followed up for 3 years (Gohel *et al.*, 2007). They found that recurrence rates were significantly lower in the compression plus surgery group compared with the compression group (31% *v.* 56%). There was also a significantly higher ulcer-free time in the compression plus surgery group. This is a useful finding, but it must be acknowledged that not all patients will be suitable for surgery because of concomitant disease.

Patients still need to be seen regularly once the ulcer is healed in order to provide encouragement and to ensure that the preventative care is understood. They should also be given information on how to get further help if the ulcer recurs. The sooner that appropriate care can be given, the sooner the ulcer will heal. Poore *et al.* (2002) monitored the impact of a healed ulcer clinic over a 2-year period. Of the 110 patients studied, 14 patients did not attend after the first year, 75 (78%) remained healed and 21 (22%) had recurrence. The authors examined the medical records to determine the actual length of time the healed ulcers had remained healed. The commonest length of time was 3 years (32%) with a range of 1.5 to 19 years.

Prevention is obviously better than cure. Ruckley *et al.* (2002) undertook a cross-sectional survey of adults aged 18–64 years randomly selected from 12 general practices. They found a 9.4% prevalence of chronic venous insufficiency in men and 6.6% in women. However, the rate rose steeply with age to 21.2% in men and 12% in women over 50 years. The research team suggest that as about one-third of the subjects had damage to the superficial veins it would be worth advocating surgical treatment to prevent leg ulceration developing at a later date.

Arterial ulcers

Aetiology

Arterial ulcers are the result of inadequate tissue perfusion to the feet or legs. This is due to complete or partial blockage of the arterial supply to the legs and the underlying condition is often referred to as peripheral vascular disease. This is a general term used to encompass disease that reduces the blood supply to the periphery. The commonest disease is arteriosclerosis where the artery walls become thickened. It is usually found in combination with atherosclerosis, the formation of plaques on the inner lining of the vessels. The lumen of the vessels gradually narrows causing ischaemia in the surrounding tissue, ultimately resulting in necrosis. This type of arterial insufficiency is most commonly found in men over the age of 50.

Buerger's disease is another type of disease affecting the peripheral arteries. Inflammation of the vessels results in thrombus formation and occlusion of the vessels. It is associated with heavy smoking and is found most commonly in men between the ages of 20 and 35 years. Ulceration associated with necrosis and gangrene may develop.

Management of arterial ulcers

Assessment

Assessment of the patient may reveal pain particularly associated with walking, intermittent claudication, that is relieved by resting. A study by Closs *et al.* (2008) assessed pain in 79 patients with leg ulcers to see if there was a difference in pain type between different aetiologies of ulcer. They found that arterial ulcers were more painful when lying down and the patients used words such as sharp, stinging or hurting to describe the pain. Those with venous ulcers described the pain as throbbing, burning or itchy. Past medical history may reveal known peripheral vascular disease or arterial surgery. A past or present history of smoking should also be noted.

When the legs are examined they may feel cold to touch and have a shiny, hairless appearance. The toe nails may be thickened and opaque. The legs become white when elevated and a reddish/blue colour when dependent. Pedal pulses are diminished or absent. Doppler examination will reveal the presence of ischaemia with an ABPI below 0.9. If the patient has intermittent claudication, the ABPI is likely to be between 0.5 and 0.9. Rest pain and an ABPI below 0.5 are indicative of critical ischaemia. The patient should be referred to a vascular surgeon.

Arterial ulcers may occur anywhere on the leg or foot but are most commonly found on the foot. The ulcer has a punched out appearance and may be deep, involving muscles or tendons. Necrosis is often present and there is often far less exudate than in venous leg ulcers, (Figure 5.3). Table 5.5 compares venous and arterial ulcers, (Dealey, 1991).

Management

Arterial ulcers are notoriously difficult to heal and arterial surgery to improve the blood supply may be necessary before an ulcer will heal. Early referral for reconstructive surgery is ideal. A systematic review considered the effects of bypass surgery for critical limb ischaemia compared with control or other treatments such as angioplasty. Despite there being large numbers of patients in the included studies the reviewers concluded there was only limited evidence to support bypass surgery compared with other treatments and more trials are required (Fowkes & Leng, 2008) Unfortunately, for some patients, despite treatment, there is

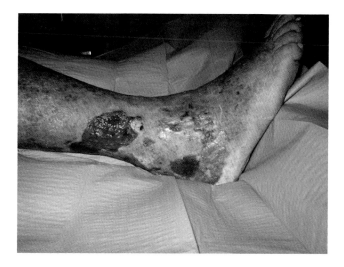

Figure 5.3 **An arterial ulcer**

considerable risk of the onset of gangrene and even septicaemia and amputation of the limb may be the only solution.

If a patient has severe resting pain, good pain control is an essential part of the management. The patient should also be encouraged to give up smoking as failure to do so will further compromise the blood supply to the leg. Gentle exercise will help to encourage the development of a collateral

Table 5.5 **A comparison of venous and arterial ulcers**

Sign/symptom	Venous ulcer	Arterial ulcer
Site	On/near medial malleolus	May be on toes, foot, heel or lateral aspect of leg
Development	Develops slowly	Develops rapidly
Appearance of ulcer	Shallow margin; deep tissues not affected	Often deep with involvement of tendons or muscles
Appearance of leg	Brown, varicose staining, and eczema, warm to touch	Shiny skin, cold to touch, white on elevation, may become blue when dependent
Oedema	Present – usually worse at end of day	Only present if patient immobile – stasis oedema
Pain	Level and time of pain varies	Very painful – worse at night. Relieved by hanging leg over side of bed
Medical history	DVT, phlebitis, varicose veins	Peripheral vascular disease, ischaemic heart disease
ABPI	0.9 and above	Below 0.9

ABPI, ankle brachial pressure index; DVT, deep vein thrombosis.

supply to the limb, thus improving tissue perfusion. The limbs should be kept warm as cold may precipitate pain.

The major aim of ulcer management is to remove necrotic tissue and to prevent infection. Selection of appropriate wound management products depends on the ulcer appearance, the amount of exudate and the position of the ulcer (see Chapters 3 and 4). A Cochrane review found only one small trial of a topical agent for arterial ulcers and concluded that there was insufficient evidence to determine whether the choice of dressing affects the healing of arterial ulcers (Nelson & Bradley, 2007).

Any dressing needs to be effectively retained and yet not so bulky as to restrict mobility unduly. Areas such as the toes are not at all easy to dress. Bandages are often needed to hold the dressing in place. Compression bandages should not be used on arterial ulcers. Comfortable retention bandages such as cotton conforming bandages are suitable. Lightweight tubular bandages can be very useful, particularly on toes. It is important to ensure that, whatever bandage is used, it does not constrict the blood supply.

Ulcers of mixed aetiology

Some patients will have both an arterial and a venous component to their ulcer. There seems to be an increase in the numbers of these types of ulcers, probably because healing rates of simple venous ulcers has improved. For example, Forssgren *et al.* (2008) found a 46% increase in the numbers of multifactorial ulcers in their 2002 prevalence survey compared with their original survey in 1988. Neequaye *et al.* (2009) in their study of 177 difficult venous leg ulcer cases found that 30% ($n = 54$) also had significant peripheral vascular disease. It is important to define the predominant factor, so that appropriate treatment may be given.

Assessment

Doppler assessment and assessment of the leg will provide an indication of the mixed aetiology. A full assessment in a vascular laboratory may be of benefit. Pain assessment, as previously discussed may also be of value.

Management

If the main factor is venous, moderate graduated compression should be worn during the day. The degree of compression should be based on patient tolerance. The WUWHS (2008) consensus document provided guidance on the levels of compression that should be used for different levels of arterial insufficiency in a mixed ulcer as well as for venous ulcers (see Table 5.6). Most patients will need to remove the compression garment at night when elevation of the legs is likely to increase ischaemic pain. Top *et al.* (2009) used a two-component system (padding and short-stretch bandages) on 24 patients with mixed aetiology ulcers and found

Table 5.6 **Guidance on the Management of mixed aetiology leg ulcers (adapted from World Union of Wound Healing Societies (2008). Reproduced by kind permission of MEP Ltd. Full document can be downloaded from www.woundsinternational.com)**

Diagnosis	Goal(s)	Treatment options	Outcomes/comments
VLU + arterial insufficiency (ABPI 0.5–0.8)	Improve perfusion	Mild to moderate compression e.g. short stretch + padding or	Arterial intervention successful: staged increase in compression; close monitoring
Risk of pressure damage and distal necrosis	Control chronic venous insufficiency and oedema	Intermittent pneumatic pump	Arterial intervention unsuccessful: advanced therapies; symptom control
	Control ischaemic pain	Arterial +/− venous intervention	
VLU + severe arterial insufficiency (ABPI <0.5)	Improve perfusion	No compression bandages or hosiery	Arterial intervention successful: staged introduction of compression; close monitoring
Risk of pressure damage, vascular occlusion, foot ulceration and infection	Control chronic venous insufficiency and oedema	Intermittent pneumatic compression only	Arterial intervention unsuccessful: advanced therapies; symptom control
	Control ischaemic pain	Urgent vascular referral, arterial investigation and intervention	
		Venous intervention when possible	

ABPI, ankle brachial pressure index; VLU, venous leg ulcer.

that it did not affect arterial blood supply. However, this was a small study and the authors did not report healing rates. Care and careful monitoring must be exercised if using compression for these patients. When arterial disease predominates, a vascular opinion must be sought. However, exercise and short periods of limb elevation can be encouraged, within the limits of patient toleration. Intermittent pneumatic compression may also be useful.

Malignant leg ulcers

A small number of leg ulcers may be malignant or have become malignant. Unfortunately the condition may be missed resulting in poor outcomes. Combemale *et al.* (2007) undertook a survey across France to identify patients who had skin cancers developing on a venous leg ulcer within the past 10 years. They identified 80 patients with 85 skin cancers of which 83 were due to squamous cell carcinoma (SCC) and 2 due to basal cell carcinoma (BCC). Local clinical signs that led to a biopsy and diagnosis were:

- abnormal granulation or overt tumour growth (65/85 cases);
- failure to heal despite appropriate treatment (11/85 cases);
- increased ulcer size despite appropriate treatment (5/85 cases);
- unusual pain (2/85cases);
- abnormal bleeding (2/85 cases).

Yang *et al.* (1996) suggest that any ulcer that fails to heal when treated appropriately should be treated as suspicious. Walsh (2002) discussed the importance of taking a biopsy from atypical ulcers or non-healing ulcers and for early referral for specialist advice.

Treatment of malignant ulcers is excision and skin grafting when caught at a reasonably early stage. Amputation may be necessary for large ulcers. Although only a small percentage of leg ulcers are malignant, it is important for nurses to be aware of the possibility and alert to the need to obtain biopsies of any atypical ulcers.

Leg ulceration in rheumatoid arthritis

It has been noted that patients with rheumatoid arthritis (RA) are more vulnerable to leg ulceration and that the aetiology is frequently multifactorial (McRorie, 2000). In a leg ulcer survey of a large inner borough of London, Moffatt *et al.* (2004) found that 35% of ulcers were multifactorial and of these 26% were associated with rheumatoid arthritis. This indicates a significant minority of patients that require careful assessment and management.

Seitz *et al.* (2010) undertook a retrospective analysis of 36 patients with RA and leg ulcers to determine the underlying factors. They found that three had necrotising vasculitis and two had pyoderma gangrenosum. Eight patients had chronic venous insufficiency, four had arterial disease and three had mixed venous and arterial aetiology. A further five patients were identified as having pressure ulcers. In 11 patients the researchers were unable to identify a cause other than restricted mobility resulting in stasis oedema and ultimately secondary lymphoedema.

Assessment

A specialist rheumatology assessment as well as a vascular assessment is required for these patients. Firth (2008) suggests that vasculitic ulcers appear suddenly and rapidly increase in size. There may be multiple ulcers that present with a punched out appearance, painful, inflamed wound margins and an indurated ulcer bed (Firth, 2008). McRorie (2000) also suggests that nutritional assessment and assessment of footwear should be undertaken.

Management

Management of these patients is complex and depends on the underlying aetiologies. Compression can be used with caution where venous disease is the dominant factor, particularly if peripheral oedema is present. A small study of 15 patients by Hafner *et al.* (2000) found that vein or arterial surgery was effective in achieving healing in 9/15 patients and markedly improving the ulcers of 5/15. They suggest a prospective trial was needed to confirm these results. Oien *et al.* (2001) used pinch grafts to treat the patients in their study group. They achieved healing in 8/20 patients, the ulcers in these patients being much smaller (range 0.4–13.2 cm^2) than the unhealed ulcers (range 6.7–356.6 cm^2). They also found a significant reduction in pain in 18/20 patients following the pinch grafting.

Summary

- Leg ulcers are painful and can have a major impact on quality of life.
- Assessment should be undertaken to determine the underlying aetiology before planning treatment.
- Compression in the mainstay of treatment for venous ulcers.
- Compression should not be used on arterial ulcers.
- Once healed, recurrence is common and surgery is increasingly being used for venous ulcers as well as arterial ulcers.
- Ulcers that do not respond to treatment may be multifactorial and further advice should be sought.

Diabetic foot ulcers

Ulceration of the foot is a serious complication of diabetes mellitus, which can lead to disability and possible amputation of the affected limb. It is extremely common with an annual incidence of 1–4% and a lifetime risk for people with diabetes developing an ulcer of about 15–25% (Snyder & Hanft, 2009). The incidence of amputation is variable, it has been shown to be between 0.5% and 1.3% in the UK, but may be as high as 7% elsewhere (Leese & Schofield, 2008).

Driver *et al.* (2010) discussed the costs of treating diabetic foot ulcers using figures from the USA. They found that about 33% of the $116 billion spent in direct costs for treating diabetes in 2007 was in relation to foot ulcers. When they compared the costs of treating diabetics with or without foot ulcers, the cost for those with foot ulcers was 5.4 times higher in the first year and 2.8 times higher in the second year. The cost is not just financial as there are higher mortality rates associated with diabetic foot ulcers. In the USA the 5-year mortality rates for those with diabetic foot ulcers or associated amputations has been shown to be 45–55%, which is higher than cancers such as prostate, breast or colon

(Armstrong *et al.*, 2007). In Norway a 10-year prospective study found that a history of diabetic foot ulcer was an independent predictor of mortality in patients with diabetes with a 38% increased risk of death (Snyder & Hanft, 2009).

Aetiology

The underlying causes of diabetic ulcers are peripheral neuropathy and peripheral vascular disease. Infection is an ever-present risk for the diabetic and can exacerbate the development of ulceration and increase the risk of amputation.

Peripheral neuropathy affects the peripheral sensory, motor and autonomic nerves of the leg. This has a two-fold effect of causing a loss of sensation and compromising the biomechanics of the foot. Muscle atrophy in the foot, particularly over the arch of the foot causes a transfer of body weight and reactive callus formation on the plantar surface. Ultimately, deformities of the foot, such as claw toes or Charcot neuro-osteoarthropathy, may occur along with alterations in gait. Peripheral neuropathy, foot deformity and trauma have been found to be the commonest combination of factors resulting in foot ulceration (Boulton, 2008). Poorly fitting shoes or a foreign body within the shoe can cause undetected injury resulting in ulcer formation. The patient may be completely unaware of the ulcer for some time.

Vascular disease in people with diabetes primarily affects the smaller arterioles within the foot. Intermittent claudication is unlikely, as larger arteries are not usually occluded. As with all types of vascular disease, it is exacerbated by smoking. Gangrene of the toes can be caused by thrombosis in the artery supplying the affected digit. Pressure from poorly fitting shoes is the commonest cause of ischaemic ulceration.

Microvascular dilatation plays a significant role in the healing of minor wounds. The ability of these vessels to dilate can be measured by using a laser Doppler to test the response to heat. A study by Sandeman *et al.* (1991) measured the ability to respond to heat by vasodilation in insulin-dependent diabetics, non-insulin-dependent diabetics and a control group of healthy individuals. A significantly worse response was found in the non-insulin-dependent diabetics than in the other two groups.

Prevention

Given the grave implications of ulceration, prevention is very important. Guidelines on the prevention and management of the diabetic foot developed by the International Working Group on the Diabetic Foot (IWGDF) suggest that there are five key elements to foot management (Apelqvist *et al.*, 2008).

(1) Regular inspection and examination of the foot at risk.
(2) Identification of the at risk foot.

(3)   Education of patient, family and healthcare providers.
(4)   Appropriate footwear.
(5)   Treatment of non-ulcerative pathology.

Regular monitoring of diabetic feet is an essential part of the guideline and should be carried out at least annually. Assessment should include: testing of foot sensation, palpation of foot pulses, inspection for any foot deformity and inspection of footwear (Apelqvist *et al.*, 2008). After assessment it is possible to classify the level of foot risk as follows:

- low current risk (normal sensation, palpable pulses);
- increased risk (neuropathy or absent pulses or other risk factor);
- high risk (neuropathy or absent pulses plus deformity or skin changes or previous ulcer);
- ulcerated foot.

Once patients have been identified as being at risk, then they should be made aware of their responsibilities for prevention of foot problems. Feet should be washed daily and dried carefully. They should be inspected for any red areas, swelling or cracked or broken skin. Toe nails should be cut straight across. Socks should be changed daily and not wrinkle. Shoes should be well fitting. They should be checked before wearing for any foreign bodies. New shoes should be properly fitted and feet carefully observed for signs of rubbing. Patients should not wear sandals or go barefoot. Those with poor vision may need assistance. Those who smoke should be encouraged to stop.

   At each attendance at the diabetic clinic, the patient should have a full foot check. This may involve the doctor, diabetic nurse specialist and podiatrist. Treatment of callus formation and management of any fungal infections is usually carried out by the podiatrist. If the patient has any deformity of the feet it may be helpful for the orthotist to assess for suitable footwear. Ill-fitting shoes is a major cause of ulceration. If the patient has other pathology requiring treatment, other health professionals should be vigilant in identifying any potential foot problems.

Management of diabetic foot ulcers

Ideally, the care of patients with diabetic foot ulcers should be within the context of a multidisciplinary foot care team comprising podiatrists, orthotists, nurses and diabetologists, all of whom should have specialist expertise in this area. NICE (2011) has provided a useful care pathway for the management of a foot problem.

Assessment

When assessing the patient there may be an indication of the type of ulcer. A history of pain associated with the ulcer, for example, almost certainly indicates ischaemia. Deformities of gait are indicative of neuropathy. Assessment of the diabetic state is important because of the increased risk of infection in the presence of hyperglycaemia.

Assessment of the leg and foot will provide objective evidence of the presence of either ischaemia or neuropathy or both. Table 5.7 indicates the differences between the two types of ulcers. However, both pathologies may be present in many patients. A survey of diabetic foot ulcer management in secondary healthcare found that 33% were neuropathic, 40% were neuro-ischaemic and 20% were ischaemic (Jude *et al.*, 2003). Vascular assessment using Doppler ultrasound can help to determine the level of ischaemia. However, it is important to be aware of the potential for a falsely elevated ABPI because of calcification of the arteries. If this is suspected, the patient should be referred for more intensive vascular assessment. An important aspect of assessment is to identify the precipitating factor. Careful assessment of footwear and the precise position of the ulcer can provide clues. It is essential to identify the cause of the ulcer, or further ulceration may occur.

Neuropathic ulcers may be surrounded by callus and have a punched-out appearance, (Figure 5.4). Ischaemic ulcers are usually covered by necrotic tissue. The ulcer should be carefully observed for any indication of infection as it poses a direct threat to the affected limb (Apelqvist *et al.*, 2008). (See also Section 2.2 in Chapter 2.)

Table 5.7   **A comparison of signs of peripheral neuropathy and peripheral vascular disease in the diabetic foot**

Sign/symptom	Neuropathic ulcer	Ischaemic ulcer
Deformity of the foot	Present as claw toe hammer toe, Charcot foot or other	Not present
Skin temperature of foot	Warm	Cold
Colour of foot	Normal	White when elevated or cyanotic
Toe nails	Atrophic	Atrophic
Pedal pulses	Present	ABPI below 0.9 (false high readings if small vessels calcified)
Pain	Present in some – associated with numbness and diminished sensation	Present, relieved by hanging legs down
Callus formation	Present, especially on plantar surface	Not present
Ulcer site	Commonly on plantar surface of foot	Commonly on toes and the edges of the foot

ABPI, ankle brachial pressure index.

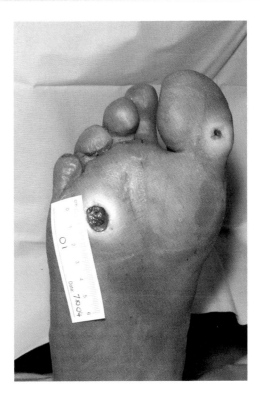

Figure 5.4   **A neuropathic ulcer**

Management

Management of diabetic foot ulcers is summarised in Table 5.8 and is based on the IWGDF guidance (Apelqvist *et al.*, 2008). Adequate control of the diabetic state is the primary goal when managing patients with foot ulceration. Pain control may also be necessary. Any callus formation should be removed regularly by a skilled healthcare professional (Bus *et al.*, 2008). Pressure must also be removed from the ulcer and this can be achieved by in several ways, although the total contact cast is the preferred treatment for non-infected neuropathic ulcers on the plantar surface of the foot (Bus *et al.*, 2008). Necrotic tissue must be debrided by use of appropriate wound management products (as discussed in Chapter 3). Any infection should be treated with systemic antibiotics and the application of suitable dressings (see Chapter 4). Compression bandages should not be used, but, if necessary, a simple retention bandage can be used to hold the dressing in place.

Some patients may benefit from revascularisation and should have a prompt referral for a vascular opinion (NICE, 2011). Faries *et al.* (2004) discussed the role of arterial reconstruction and noted that in centres

Table 5.8   **Summary of International Working Group on the Diabetic Foot guidelines for managing diabetic foot ulcers (based on Apelqvist *et al.*, 2008)**

Principle	Comment
Relief of pressure and ulcer protection	Offloading preferably by total contact cast, but other alternatives included removable walkers or cast shoes
Restoration of skin perfusion	Mainly by angioplasty or bypass surgery. However, attention should be paid to smoking cessation and treatment of hypertension
Treatment of infection	Treatment of local infection by debridement and oral antibiotics Deep infection requires immediate surgical drainage $+/-$ removal of necrotic tissue and infected bone
Metabolic control	Optimal diabetes control reduces risk of infection
Local wound care	See Chapters 3 and 4
Education	Patients should understand principles of management, undertake self-care as appropriate and be able to report signs and symptoms of infection
Prevention of recurrence	Understanding the initial cause is essential for future prevention Patient should be enrolled onto a life-long comprehensive foot care programme

of excellence 70% of surgical bypass grafts will still be patent after 5 years and the associated 5-year limb-salvage rate was greater than 80%.

Once the ulcer is healed, preventative measures need to be instigated including patient and family education, review of footwear and swift access to care in the event of further problems.

The management of fungating wounds

Malignant fungating wounds are particularly difficult wounds to manage. They are distressing for both the sufferer and the nurse. Although the literature is gradually increasing, there is still a paucity of evidence to guide practice. It is undoubtedly a difficult area to research, but it is an important area to tackle, not least in order to improve the quality of life for these patients.

Aetiology and incidence

Fungating lesions occur when a cancerous mass invades the epithelium, thus ulcerating through to the body surface. There is little epidemiological evidence, but Alexander (2009a) suggests that it is reasonable to predict that over 5% of cancer patients will develop a malignant wound. This is supported by a Swiss survey of oncology nurses who reported a prevalence of 6.6% in their patient group (Probst *et al.*, 2009). Fungating wounds most commonly occur with cancer of the breast, but may also be found in cancers of the skin, head and neck, vulva and bladder (Dowsett, 2002). Fungating wounds not only develop at the site of the primary tumour, but if the nodes of the groin or axilla are affected, ulceration may also occur at that site. Fungating wounds can grow rapidly and cause massive skin damage (Alexander, 2009a).

Impact on quality of life

A fungating wound can have a devastating effect on the sufferer. Lo *et al.* (2008) interviewed 10 patients and identified a number of themes in the analysis that included declining physical well-being and wound-related stigma. Within the theme of declining physical well-being were subthemes of: wound pain, wound odour and wound exudate. The wound-related symptoms resulted in distress, embarrassment and ultimately social isolation.

Piggin and Jones (2007) undertook a small study of five participants and found these wounds had a similar impact in their study. They found that the physical problems caused by the wound were the worst part of the cancer, especially because of the vulnerability of not knowing if it would leak or bleed or the odour become obvious to others. As a result it changed their relationships with others and they felt a loss of identity, while striving to be normal.

The Lo *et al.* (2008) study does have a positive outcome in that once they received help from the wound nurse specialist they found that their symptoms were better managed. The fact that they no longer had to deal with pain, leakage and odour, enabled the patients to regain self-confidence and they no longer withdrew from their family and friends. Although these are only small studies, there is value in learning from the patient perspective.

Management of fungating wounds

Grocott (2007) suggested this can be divided into:

- treatment of the underlying tumour and management of comorbidities;
- symptom management;
- local wound management.

Treatment of the underlying tumour is beyond the scope of this book. Symptom management includes the management of pain and psychosocial issues and these have discussed in Chapter 2.

Local wound management

Chapter 3 covers the general principles of wound management. This section will address the specific problems related to fungating wounds.

Assessment

When assessing the wound the following need to be considered.

- Fungating lesions are often necrotic, sloughy or infected.
- There is usually copious amounts of exudate, which may have an offensive odour.
- Many of these wounds become malodorous as a result of bacterial invasion. It causes distress to the patient, relatives and visitors. It may be very difficult to control.
- The position of the wound obviously depends of the type of cancer. However, it may spread along the trunk or limbs, sometimes in the form of isolated nodules. Applying a dressing to protect such a spread out lesion can be very difficult and requires considerable nursing skill.
- Capillary bleeding may occur as the cancer increases in size and erodes blood vessels. It may be sufficiently heavy or frequent to cause anaemia. Removal of the old dressing must be done with great care in order to avoid loosening any clots.

Alexander (2009a) has provided a useful framework for wound assessment.

Management

It is essential to identify patient problems rather than nurse problems. While in many instances they may be the same, they are not always. Once the specific problems have been identified, the treatment options have to be planned in the light of the patient's condition. If the expected outcome is very poor, then totally palliative care with the minimum need to dress the wound must be the treatment of choice. For others, a more aggressive approach can be used. A course of radiotherapy may be prescribed to help reduce the size of the lesion. It should be remembered that many patients find dressing change a major ordeal that leaves them feeling very tired.

Bleeding: capillary bleeding can be frightening for both the patient and the nurse. When there is a history of capillary bleeding, great care should be taken when removing the old dressing. If the dressing is adherent, it should be soaked with saline before removal is attempted. It may also be necessary to remove the dressing slowly in stages. It is better to take a long time to remove a dressing than to start bleeding that is difficult to control. Gentle irrigation using a syringe can be helpful in removing loose debris.

There is little evidence to guide clinical practice and what there is anecdotal (Alexander, 2009b). Adrenaline can be applied directly to the wound to control profuse bleeding. However, it should be used with caution, under medical supervision. Alginate dressings are useful when there is oozing. They can be removed easily by washing away with saline. Haemostatic surgical sponges have also been used successfully. If there is persistent bleeding, the haemoglobin should be checked regularly. Blood transfusions may be necessary to treat anaemia.

Exudate: as previously noted copious exudate is problem that concerns patients. Alexander (2009c) reviewed the problems in managing exudate and the lack of specific dressings for this wound type and found that often two or more dressing layers are used. She suggests that the primary layer should be non-adherent, conformable and able to vent moisture to the secondary layer. It should also be possible to remove this layer without causing trauma. The secondary layer dressing should be conformable, highly absorbent and as aesthetically acceptable as possible. Grocott (1997 & 1998) has undertaken a longitudinal multiple case study design to monitor the outcomes when using different dressings to manage exudate. She considered that the factor of greatest importance is fitting conformable dressing materials to the wound, thus reducing the risk of leakage. Dressing bulk can be reduced by the use of outer dressings with high moisture vapour transfer rates. Hydrofibres, alginates and hydrocellular foams can be effective in controlling exudate.

Odour: this causes great distress to patients. It is mostly due to bacterial invasion, although exuding necrotic wounds may also be offensive. A wound swab will identify the invading bacteria, so that appropriate systemic antibiotics can be prescribed. Topical agents can also be used. Costa Santos *et al.* (2010) undertook a systematic review to determine effective management of odour, but they only found a small number of poorly described studies. The review team found some evidence that topical metronidazole could reduce odour. There was also limited evidence for the use of Mesalt® (an absorbent viscose material impregnated with sodium chloride) or activated carbon dressings. Silver, honey and iodine dressings have also been described in the literature as well as the use of essential oils such as eucalyptus, tea tree or lemon myrtle (Alexander, 2009c).

When aggressive treatment is suitable, wound debridement is a treatment option. Removal of necrotic or sloughy tissue can reduce odour and exudate. The quickest method is surgical debridement. This must be done by a skilled surgeon because of the distorted anatomy and the risk of capillary bleeding. Surgical debridement is not a suitable option for patients with a history of capillary bleeding into the wound.

Conclusions

Managing fungating wounds is extremely challenging and the focus should be on addressing the patient's problems. However, if a dressing regime can be identified that controls odour and exudate and is comfortable to wear and does not cause trauma at dressing change then it is possible to make a major difference to a patient's quality of life.

Conclusion to chapter 5

The management of chronic wounds is complex and requires skilled care that is best undertaken with a multiprofessional team. Fortunately, there is increasing access to specialist services that have a made a major impact and improvement in patient care.

References

Alexander S (2009a) Malignant fungating wounds: epidemiology, aetiology, presentation and assessment. *Journal of Wound Care*, **18**: 273–280.

Alexander S (2009b) Malignant fungating wounds: managing pain, bleeding and psychosocial issues. *Journal of Wound Care*, **18**: 418–425.

Alexander S (2009c) Malignant fungating wounds: managing malodour and exudate. *Journal of Wound Care*, **18**: 374–382.

Amsler F, Willenberg T, Blattler W (2009) In search of optimal compression therapy for venous leg ulcers: a meta-analysis of studies comparing diverse bandages with specifically designed stockings. *Journal of Vascular Surgery*, **50**: 668–674.

Apelqvist J, Bakker K, van Houtum WH, Schaper (2008) Practical guidelines on the management and prevention of the diabetic foot. Based upon the International Consensus of the Diabetic Foot (2007). Prepared by the International Working Group on the Diabetic Foot. *Diabetes/Metabolism Research & Reviews*, **24** (suppl 1): S181–S187.

Armstrong DG, Wrobel J, Robbins JM (2007) Guest editorial: are diabetes-related wounds and amputations worse than cancer? *International Wound Journal*, **4**: 286–287.

Banks M, Bauer J, Graves N, Ash S (2010) Malnutrition and pressure ulcer risk in adults in Australian health care facilities. *Nutrition*, **26**: 896–901.

Bates-Jenson, Early L, Seeman S (2004) Skin Disorders. In: Ferrell BR, Coyle N, eds. *Textbook of Palliative Nursing*, 2nd edn. New York: Oxford University Press Inc, pp. 301–328.

Beeckman D, Schoonhoven L, Verhaeghe, Heyneman A, Defloor T (2009) Prevention and treatment of incontinence-associated dermatitis. *Journal of Advanced Nursing*, **65**: 1141–1154.

Bergstrom N, Braden B, Brandt J, Krall K (1985) Adequacy of descriptive scales for reporting diet intake in the institutionalised elderly. *Journal of Nutrition for the Elderly*, **6**: 3–16.

Bergstrom N, Braden B, Laguzza A (1987) The Braden scale for predicting pressure sore risk. *Nursing Research*, **36**: 205–210.

Bergstrom N, Braden B, Kemp M, Champagne M, Ruby E (1996) Multi-site study of incidence of pressure ulcers and the relationship between risk level, demographic characteristics, diagnoses and prescription of preventive interventions. *Journal of the American Geriatric Society*, **44**: 22–30.

Bliss M (1990) Editorial - preventing pressure sores. *Lancet*, **335**: 1311–1312.

Bou JE, Segovia GT, Verdu SJ, Nolasco BA, Rueda LJ, Perejamo M (2005) The effectiveness of a hyperoxygenated fatty acid compound in preventing pressure ulcers. *Journal of Wound Care*, **14**: 117–121.

Boulton AJM (2008) The diabetic foot: grand overview, epidemiology and pathogenesis. *Diabetes/Metabolism Research & Reviews*, **24** (suppl 1): S3–S6.

Boyle M, Green M (2001) Pressure sores in intensive care: defining their incidence and associated factors and assessing the utility of two pressure sore risk assessment tools. *Australian Critical Care*, **14**: 24–30.

Briggs M, Closs SJ (2003) The prevalence of leg ulceration: a review of the literature. *EWMA Journal*, **3**: 14–20.

Branski LK, Gauglitz GG, Herndon DN, Jeschke MG. (2009) A review of gene and stem cell therapy in cutaneous wound healing. *Burns*, **35**: 171–180.

Bus SA, Valk GD, Armstrong DG, Caravaggi C, Hlaváček P, Bakker K, Cavanagh PR (2008) Specific guidelines on footwear and offloading. *Diabetes/Metabolism Research & Reviews*, **24** (suppl 1): S192–S193.

Buss IC, Halfens RJ, Abu-Saad HH (1997) The effectiveness of massage in preventing pressure sores: a literature review. *Rehabilitation Nursing*, **22**: 229–234.

Cadue JF, Karolewicz S, Tardy C, BarraultC, Robert R, Pourrat O (2008) Prevention of heel pressure sores with a foam body-support device. A randomised controlled trial in a medical intensive care unit. *Presse Medicine*, **37**: 30–36.

Cameron, J. (1998) Skin care for patients with chronic leg ulcers. *Journal of Wound Care*, **7**: 459–462.

Clark M, Bours G, Defloor T (2003) The prevalence of pressure ulcers in Europe. *Hospital Decisions*, **Winter 2003/2004**: 123–129.

Clark M, Romanelli M, Reger SI, Ranganathan VK, Black J, Dealey C (2010) Microlclimate in context. In: *InternationalReview: Pressure Ulcer Prevention: Pressure, Shear, Friction and Microclimate. A Consensus Document*. London: Wounds International, pp. 19–25.

Closs SJ, Nelson EA, Briggs M (2008) Can venous and arterial leg ulcers be differentiated by the characteristics of the pain they produce? *Journal of Clinical Nursing*, **17**: 637–645.

Collins F (1999) The contribution made by an armchair with integral pressure-reducing cushion in the prevention of pressure sore incidence in the elderly, acutely ill patient. *Journal of Tissue Viability*, **9**: 133–137.

Combemale P. Bousquet M. Kanitakis J. Bernard P. (2007) Malignant transformation of leg ulcers: a retrospective study of 85 cases. *Journal of the European Academy of Dermatology & Venereology*, **21**: 935–41.

Connor T, Sledge JA, Bryant-Wiersema L, Stamm L, Potter P (2010) Identification of pre-operative and intra-operative variables predictive of pressure ulcer development in patients undergoing urologic surgical procedures. *Urologic Nursing*, **30**: 289–295, 305.

Costa Santos CM, Mattos Pimenta CA, Nobre MRC (2010) A systematic review of topical treatments to control the odour of malignant fungating wounds. *Journal of Pain & Symptom Management*, **39**: 1065–1076.

David JA, Chapman RG, Chapman EJ, Lockett B (1983) *An investigation of the current methods used in nursing for the care of patients with established pressure sores*. Northwick Park, Middlesex: Nursing Practice Research Unit.

Dealey C (1991) Causes of leg ulcers. *Nursing*, **4**: 23–24.

Dealey C (1997) *Managing Pressure Sore Prevention*. Salisbury: Mark Allen Publishing.

Defloor T, Schoonhoven L (2004) Interrater reliability of the EPUAP pressure ulcer classification system using photographs. *Journal of Clinical Nursing*, **13**: 952–959.

Defloor T, de Bacquer D, Grypdonck (2005) The effect of various combinations of turning and pressure reducing devices on the incidence of pressure ulcers. *International Journal of Nursing Studies*, **42**: 37–46.

Defloor T, Grypdonck MFH (2005) Pressure ulcers: validation of two risk assessment scales. *Journal of Clinical Nursing*, **14**: 373–382.

Defloor T, Schoonhoven L, Vanderwee K, Westrate J (2006) Reliability of the European Pressure Ulcer Advisory Panel classification system. *Journal of Advanced Nursing*, **54**: 189–198.

Department of Health (2010) *The NHS Outcomes Framework 2011/12*. London: Department of Health.

Dowsett C (2002) Malignant fungating wounds: assessment and management. *British Journal of Community Nursing*, **7**: 394–400.

Driver VR, Fabbi M, Lavery LA, Gibbons G (2010) The costs of diabetic foot: the economic case for the limb salvage team. *Journal of the American Podiatric Medical Association*, **100**: 335–341.

Dumville JC, Worthy G, Soares MO, Bland JM, Cullum N, Dowson C, Iglesias C, McCaughan D, Nelson EA, Torgerson D (2009) Venus II: a randomised controlled trial in the management of leg ulcers. *Health Technology Assessment*, **13**: 1–182.

Ek AC, Gustavssen G, Lewis DH (1987) Skin blood flow in relation to external pressure and temperature in the supine position on a standard hospital mattress. *Scandinavian Journal of Rehabilitation*, **19**: 121–126.

Exton-Smith AN, Sherwin RW (1961) The prevention of pressure sores: the significance of spontaneous bodily movement. *Lancet*, **II**: 1124–1126.

Faries PL, Teodorescu VJ, Morrissey NJ, Hollier LH, Marin ML (2004) The role of surgical revascularisation in the management of diabetic foot wounds. *American Journal of Surgery*, **187** (suppl): 34S–37S.

Finlayson K, Edwards H, Courtney M (2009) Factors associated with recurrence of venous ulcers: a survey and retrospective chart review. *International Journal of Nursing Studies*, **46**: 1071–1078.

Finlayson K, Edwards H, Courtney M (2010) The impact of psychosocial factors on adherence to compression therapy to prevent recurrence of venous leg ulcers. *Journal of Clinical Nursing*, **19**: 1289–1297.

Firth J (2008) Lower limb ulceration in rheumatoid arthritis. *Nursing Times*, **104**: 40–42.

Firth J, Nelson EA, Hale C, Hill J, Helliwell P (2010) A review of design and reporting issues in self-reported prevalence studies of leg ulceration. *Journal of Clinical Epidemiology*, **63**: 907–913.

Fogerty MD, Abumrad NN, Nanney L, Argobast PG, Poulose B, Barbul A (2008) Risk factors for pressure ulcers in acute care hospitals. *Wound Repair & Regeneration*, **16**: 11–18.

Forssgren A, Fransson I, Nelzen O (2008) Leg ulcer point prevalence can be decreased by broad-scale intervention: a follow-up cross-sectional study of a defined geographical population. *Acta Dermato-Venereologica*, **88**: 252–256.

Fowks F, Leng GG (2008) Bypass surgery for chronic lower limb ischaemia. *Cochrane Database of Systematic Reviews*, **2**: CD002000..

Frankel H, Sperry J, Kaplan L (2007) Risk factors for pressure ulcer development in a best practice surgical intensive care unit. *The American Surgeon*, **73**: 1215–1217.

Friedberg EH, Harrison MB, Graham ID (2002) Current home care expenditure for persons with leg ulcers. *Journal of Wound, Ostomy & Continence Nursing*, **29**: 186–192.

Gebhardt, K, Bliss M (1994) Preventing pressure sores in orthopaedic patients. Is prolonged chair sitting detrimental? *Journal of Tissue Viability*, **4**: 51–54.

Gohel MS, Barwell JR, Taylor M, Chant T, Foy C, Earnshaw JJ, Heather BP, Mitchell DC, Whyman MR, Poskitt KR (2007) Long term results of compression therapy alone versus compression plus surgery in chronic venous ulceration (ESCHAR): randomised controlled trial. *British Medical Journal*, **335**: 83–88.

Gorecki C, Brown JM, Nelson EA, Briggs M, Schoonhoven L, Dealey C, Defloor T, Nixon J (2009) Impact of pressure ulcers on quality of life in older patients: a systematic review. *Journal of the American Geriatric Society*, **57**: 1175–1183.

Graham ID, Harrison MB, Nelson EA, Lorimer K, Fisher A (2003) Prevalence of lower limb ulceration: a systematic review of prevalence studies. *Advances in Skin & Wound Care*, **16**: 305–316.

Grocott P (1997) Evaluation of a tool to assess the management of fungating wounds. *Journal of Wound Care*, **6**: 421–424.

Grocott P (1998) Exudate management in fungating wounds. *Journal of Wound Care*, **7**: 445–448.

Grocott P (2007) Care of patients with fungating malignant wounds. *Nursing Standard*, **21**: 57–64.

Hafner J, Schneider E, Burg G, Cassina PC (2000) Management of leg ulcers in patients with rheumatoid arthritis or systemic sclerosis: the importance of concomitant arterial and venous disease. *Journal of Vascular Surgery*, **32**: 322–329.

Haglsawa S, Barbenel J (1999) The limits of pressure sore prevention. *Journal of the Royal Society of Medicine*, **92**: 576–578.

Heyneman A, Beele H, Vanderwee K, Defloor T (2008) A systematic review of the use of hydrocolloids in the treatment of pressure ulcers. *Journal of Clinical Nursing*, **17**: 1164–1173.

Hofman D, Ryan TJ, Arnold F, Cherry GW, Lindholm C, Bjellerup M, Glynn C (1997) Pain in venous leg ulcers. *Journal of Wound Care*, **6**: 222–224.

Hopkins A, Dealey C, Bale S, Defloor T, Worboys F (2006) Patient stories of living with a pressure ulcer. *Journal of Advanced Nursing*, **56**: 345–353.

James J, Evans JA, Young T, Clark M (2010) Pressure ulcer prevalence across Welsh orthopaedic units and community hospitals: surveys based on the European Pressure Ulcer Advisory Panel minimum data set. *International Wound Journal*, **7**: 147–152.

Jones JE, Nelson EA (2007) Skin grafting for venous leg ulcers. *Cochrane Database of Systematic Reviews*, **2**: CD001737.

Jones JE, Robinson J, Barr W, Carlisle C (2008) Impact of exudate and odour from chronic venous leg ulceration. *Nursing Standard*, **22**: 53–61.

Jude EB, Oyibo SO, Millichip MM, Boulton AJM (2003) A survey of physicians' involvement in the management of diabetic foot ulcers in secondary health care. *Practical Diabetes International*, **20**: 89–92.

Jull A, Arroll B, Parag V, Waters J (2007) Pentoxifylline for treating venous leg ulcers. *Cochrane Database of Systematic Reviews*, **3**, CD001733.

Jull A, Parag V, Walker N, Maddison R, Kerse N, Johns T (2009) The PREPARE pilot RCT of home-based progressive resistance exercises for venous leg ulcers. *Journal of Wound Care*, **18**: 497–503.

Kan YM, Delis KT (2001) Haemodynamic effects of supervised calf muscle exercise in patients with venous ulceration. *Archives of Surgery*, **136**: 1364–1369.

Keys KA, Daniali LN, Warner KJ, Mathes DW (2010) multivariate predictors of failure after flap coverage of pressure ulcers. *Plastic & Reconstructive Surgery*, **125**: 1725–1734.

Kierney PC, Engrav LH, Isik FF, Esselman PC, Cardenas DD, Rand RP (1998) Results of 268 pressure sores in 158 patients managed jointly by plastic surgery and rehabilitation medicine. *Plastic & Reconstructive Surgery*, **102**: 765–772.

Krapfl LE, Gray M (2008) Does regular repositioning prevent pressure ulcers? *Journal of Wound, Ostomy & Continence Nursing*, **35**: 571–577.

Krouskop M (1983) A synthesis of the factors which contribute to pressure sore formation. *Medical Hypothesis*, **11**: 255–267.

Lahmann NA, Dassen T, Poehler A, Kottner J (2010) Pressure ulcer prevalence rates from 2002 – 2008 in German long-term care facilities. *Ageing Clinical and Experimental Research*, **22**: 152–156.

Landis EM (1931) Micro-injection studies of capillary blood pressure in human skin. *Heart*, **15**: 209–228.

Langer G, Schloemer G, Knerr A, Kuss O, Behrens J (2003) Nutritional interventions for preventing and treating pressure ulcers. *Cochrane Database of Systematic Reviews*, **4**: CD003216..

Leese GP, Schofield CJ (2008) Amputations in diabetes: a changing scene. *Practical Diabetes International*, **25**: 297–299.

Lingren M, Unosson M, Fredrikson M, Ek E-C (2004) Immobility – a major risk factor for development of pressure ulcers among adult hospitalised patients: a prospective study. *Scandinavian Journal of Caring Sciences*, **18**: 57–64.

Lingren M, Unosson M, Krantz A-M, Ek E-C (2005) Pressure ulcer risk in patients undergoing surgery. *Journal of Advanced Nursing*, **50**: 605–612.

Lizaka S, Okuwa M, Sugama J, Sanada M (2010) The impact of malnutrition and nutrition-related factors on the development and severity of pressure ulcers in older patients receiving home care. *Clinical Nutrition*, **29**: 47–53.

Lo S-F, Hu W-Y, Hayter M, Chang S-C, Hsu M-y, Wu L-y (2008) Experiences of living with a malignant fungating wound: a qualitative study. *Journal of Clinical Nursing*, **17**: 2699–2708.

Lohi J, Sipponen A, Jokinen JJ (2010) Local dressings for pressure ulcers: what is the best tool to apply in primary and second care? *Journal of Wound Care*, **19**: 123–127.

Machet L, Couhe C, Perrinaud A, Hoarau C, Lorette G, Vaillant L (2004) A high prevalence of sensitisation still persists in leg ulcer patients: a retrospective series of 106 patients tested between 2001 and 2002 and a meta-analysis of 1975–2003 data. *British Journal of Dermatology*, **150**: 929–935.

Margolis DJ, Berlin JA, Strom BL (2000) Which venous leg ulcers will heal with limb compression bandages? *American Journal of Medicine*, **109**: 15–19.

Margolis D, Knauss J, Bilker W, Baumgarten M (2003) Medical conditions as risk factors for pressure ulcers in an out-patient setting. *Age & Ageing*, **32**: 259–264.

Marston W, Vowden K (2003) Compression therapy: a guide to safe practice. *EWMA Position Document: Understanding Compression Therapy*. London: Medical Education Partnership Ltd, pp. 11–17.

Mathus-Vliegen EMH (2001) Nutritional status, nutrition and pressure ulcers. *Nutrition in Clinical Practice*, **16**: 286–291.

McCafferty E, Watret L, Brown C (2000) A multidisciplinary audit of patients' seating needs. *Professional Nurse*, **15**: 715–718.

McInnes E, Cullum NA, Bell-Syer SEM, Dumville JC, Jammali-Blasi A. (2008) Support surfaces for pressure ulcer prevention. *Cochrane Database of Systematic Reviews*, **4**: CD001735.

McRorie ER (2000) The management and assessment of leg ulcers in rheumatoid arthritis. *Journal of Wound Care*, **9**: 289–292.

Medical Education Partnership (2009) *International Guidelines Pressure Ulcer Prevention: Prevalence and Incidence in Context*. London: MEP Ltd.

Moffatt CJ, Franks PJ, Doherty DC, Martin R, Blewitt R, Ross F (2004) Prevalence of leg ulceration in a London population. *Quarterly Journal of Medicine*, **97**: 431–437.

Moffatt C, Konnala D, Dourdin N, Choe Y (2009) Venous leg ulcers: patient concordance with compression therapy and its impact on healing and prevention of recurrence. *International Wound Journal*, **6**: 386–393.

Moore ZEH, Cowman S (2008) Risk assessment tools for the prevention of pressure ulcers. *Cochrane Database of Systematic Reviews*, **3**: CD006471.

Mustoe TA, O'Shaughnessy K, Kloeters O (2006) Chronic wound pathogenesis and current treatment strategies: a unifying hypothesis. *Journal of Plasic & Reconstructive Surgery*, **117**: 35–41..

National Institute for Clinical Excellence (2011) *Clinical Guideline 119: Diabetic Foot Problems*. London: NICE.

National Pressure Ulcer Advisory Panel (2007) *Support Surface Standards Initiative – Terms and Definitions Related to Support Surfaces*. Washington DC: NPUAP.

National Pressure Ulcer Advisory Panel (2010) *Not all Pressure Ulcers are Avoidable*. Washington DC: NPUAP (http://www.npuap.org/A_UA% 20Press%20Release.pdf).

National Pressure Ulcer Advisory Panel/European Pressure Ulcer Advisory Panel (2009) *Prevention and Treatment of Pressure Ulcers: Clinical Practice Guideline*. Washington DC: NPUAP.

Neequaye SK, Douglas AD, Hofman D, Wolz M, Sharma R, Cummings R, Hands L (2009) The difficult venous ulcer: case series of 177 ulcers referred for vascular surgical opinion following failure of conservative management. *Angiology*, **60**: 492–495.

Nelson EA, Bradley MD (2007) Dressings and topical agents for arterial leg ulcers. *Cochrane Database of Systematic Reviews*, **1**: CD001836.

Nelson EA, Bell-Syer SEM, Cullum NA, Webster J (2010) Compression for preventing recurrence of venous ulcers (Review). *The Cochrane Database of Systematic Reviews*, **4**: CD002303.

Nelson EA, Mani R, Vowden K (2008) Intermittent pneumatic compression for treating venous leg ulcers. *Cochrane Database of Systematic Reviews*, **2**: CD001899.

Nelzen O, Bergqvist D, Fransson I, Lindhagen A (1996a) Prevalence and aetiology of leg ulcers in a defined population of industrial workers. *Phlebology*, **11**: 50–54.

Nelzen O, Bergqvist D, Lindhagen A (1996b) the prevalence of chronic lower limb ulceration has been underestimated: results of a validated population questionnaire. *British Journal of Surgery*, **83**: 255–258.

NHS Institute for Innovation and Improvement (2008) *Commissioning for Quality and Innovation (CQUIN) Payment Framework*. London: Department of Health (http://www.institute.nhs.uk/world_class_commissioning/pct_portal/cquin.html).

Nixon J, Nelson EA, Cranny G, Iglesias CP, Hawkins K, Cullum NA, Phillips A, Spilsbury K, Torgerson DJ, Mason S (2006) Pressure relieving support surfaces: a randomised evaluation. *Health Technology Assessment*, **10**: 1–177.

Nixon J, Cranny G, Bond S (2007) Skin alterations of intact skin and risk factors associated with pressure ulcer development in surgical patients: a cohort study. *International Journal of Nursing Studies*, **44**: 655–663.

Norton D, Mclaren R, Exton-Smith AN (1975) *An Investigation of Geriatric Nursing Problems*. Edinburgh: Churchill Livingstone.

Nyquist R, Hawthorn PJ (1987) The prevalence of pressure sores in an area health authority. *Journal of Advanced Nursing*, **12**: 183–187.

O'Brien JF, Grace PA, Perry IJ, Burke PE (2000) Prevalence and aetiology of leg ulcers in Ireland. *Irish Journal of Medical Science*, **169**: 110–112.

Oien RF, Hakansson A, Hansen BU (2001) Leg ulcers in patients with rheumatoid arthritis – a prospective study of aetiology, wound healing and pain reduction after pinch grafting. *Rheumatology*, **40**: 816–820.

O'Meara S, Cullum NA, Nelson EA (2009) Compression for venous leg ulcers. *Cochrane Database of Systematic Reviews*, **1**: CD000265.

Orsted H, Rosenthal S, Woodbury MG (2009) Pressure ulcer awareness and prevention programme: a quality improvement programme through the Canadian Association of Wound Care. *Journal of Wound, Ostomy & Continence Nursing*, **36**: 178–183.

Palfreyman SSJ, Nelson EA, Lochiel R, Michaels JA (2010) Dressings for healing venous leg ulcers. *Cochrane Database of Systematic Reviews*, **3**: CD001103.

Patton LR (2009) Are community leg ulcer clinics more cost-effective than home care visits? *Journal of Wound Care*, **18**: 49–52.

Payne WG, Posnett J, Alvarez O, Brown-Etris M, Jameson G, Wolcott W, Dharma H, Hartwell S, Ochs D (2009) A prospective randomised clinical trial to assess the cost-effectiveness of a modern foam dressing vs a traditi9nal saline. *Ostomy Wound Management*, **55**: 50–55.

Persoon A, Heinen MM, van der Vleuten CJM, de Rooij MJ, van de Kerkhof PCM, van Achterberg T (2004) Leg ulcers: a review of their impact on daily life. *Journal of Clinical Nursing*, **13**: 341–354.

Piggin C, Jones V (2007) Malignant fungating wounds: an analysis of the lived experience. *International Journal of Palliative Nursing*, **13**: 384–391.

Poore S, Cameron J, Cherry G (2002) Venous leg ulcer recurrence: prevention and healing. *Journal of Wound Care*, **11**: 197–199.

Posnett J, Franks PJ (2007) The costs of skin breakdown and ulceration in the UK. In: Pownall M ed. *Skin Breakdown: The Silent Epidemic*. Hull: Smith & Nephew Foundation.

Preston KW (1988) Positioning for comfort and pressure relief: the 30 degree alternative. *Care - Science and Practice*, **6**: 116–119.

Probst S, Arber A, Faithfull S (2009) Malignant fungating wounds: a survey of nurses' clinical practice in Switzerland. *European Journal of Oncology Nursing*, **13**: 295–298.

Purwins S, Herberger K, Debus ES, Rustenbach SJ, Pelzer P, Rabe E, Schäfer E, Stadler R, Augustin M (2010) Cot-of-illness ofchronic leg ulcers in Germany. *International Wound Journal*, **7**: 97–102.

Reger SI, Ranganathan VK, Orsted HL, Ohura T, Gefen A (2010) Shear and friction in context. In: *InternationalReview: Pressure Ulcer Prevention: Pressure, Shear, Friction and Microclimate. A Consensus Document*. London: Wounds International, pp. 11–18.

Rich SE, Margolis D, Shardell M, Hawkes WG, Miller RR, Amr S, Baumgarten M (2011) Frequent repositioning and incidence of pressure ulcers among bed-bound elderly hip fracture patients. *Wound Repair & Regeneration*, **19**: 10–18.

Rithalia SVS (1989) Comparison of pressure distribution in wheelchair seat cushions. *Care - Science & Practice*, **7**: 87–89.

Royal College of Nursing (2003) *Safer Staff, Better Care: RCN Manual Handling Training Guidance and Competencies*. London: Royal College of Nursing.

Ruckley CV, Evans CJ, Allan PL, Lee AJ, Fowkes F, Gerald R (2002) Chronic venous insufficiency: clinical and duplex correlations. The Edinburgh Vein Study of venous disorders in the general population. *Journal of Vascular Surgery*, **36**: 52–525.

Ryan TJ (1987) *The Management of Leg Ulcers*, 2nd edn. Oxford: Oxford University Press.

Sanada H, Miyachi Y, Ohura T, Moriguchi T, Tokunaga K, Shido K, Nakagami G (2008) The Japanese pressure ulcer surveillance study: a retrospective cohort study to determine prevalence of pressure ulcers in Japan. *Wounds*, **20**: 20–26.

Sandeman DD, Pym CA, Green EM, Seamark C, Shore AC Tooke JE (1991) Microvascular vasodilation in the feet of newly diagnosed non-insulin dependent diabetics. *British Medical Journal*, **302**: 1122–1123.

Scanlon E, Stubbs N (2004) Pressure ulcer risk assessment in patients with darkly pigmented skin. *Professional Nurse*, **19**: 339–341.

Schoonhoven L, Defloor T, Grypdonck MH (2002a) Incidence of pressure ulcers due to surgery. *Journal of Clinical Nursing*, **11**: 479–487.

Schoonhoven L, Haalboom JRE, Bousema T, Algra A, Grobbee DE, Grypdonck MH, Burskens E (2002b) Prospective cohort study of routine use of risk assessment scales for prediction of pressure ulcers. *British Medical Journal*, **325**: 797–801.

Schoonhoven L, Grobee DE, Donders ART, Algra A, Grypdonck MH, Bousema MT, Schrijvers AJP, Buskens E (2006) Prediction of pressure ulcer development in hospitalised patients: a tool for risk assessment. *Quality & Safety in Health Care*, **15**: 65–70.

Scottish Intercollegiate Guideline Network (2010) *Management of Chronic Venous Leg Ulcers. A National Clinical Guideline*. Edinburgh: SIGN.

Seitz CS, Berens N, Bröcker E-B, Trautman A (2010) Leg ulceration in rheumatoid arthritis – an underreported multicausal complication with considerable morbidity: analysis of thirty-six patients and review of the literature. *Dermatology*, **220**: 268–273.

Sibbald RG, Krasner DL, Lutz J. (2010) SCALE: Skin Changes at Life's End: final consensus statement: October 1, 2009. *Advances in Skin & Wound Care*, **23**: 225–36.

Singh R, Singh R, Rohilla RK, Siwach R, Verma V, Kaur K (2010) Surgery for pressure ulcers improves general health and quality of life in patients with spinal cord injury. *Journal of Spinal Cord Medicine*, **33**: 396–400.

Snyder RJ, Hanft JR (2009) Diabetic foot ulcers – effects on quality of life, costs, and mortality and the role of standard wound care and advanced care therapies in healing: a review. *Ostomy Wound Management*, **55**: 28–38.

Sorensen JL, Jorgensen B, Gottrup F (2004) Surgical treatment of pressure ulcers. *American Journal of Surgery*, **188** (suppl): 42–51.

Spilsbury K, Nelson EA, Cullum N, Iglesias C, Nixon J, Mason S (2007) Pressure ulcers and their treatment and effects on quality of life: hospital inpatient perspectives. *Journal of Advanced Nursing*, **57**: 494–504.

Spittle M, Collins RJ, Connor H (2001) The incidence of pressure sores following lower limb amputations. *Practical Diabetes International*, **18**: 57–61.

Srivastava A, Gupta A, Taly AB, Murali T (2009) Surgical management of pressure ulcers during inpatient neurological rehabilitation: outcomes for patients with spinal cord disease. *Journal of Spinal Cord Medicine*, **32**: 125–131.

Stemmer R (1969) Ambulatory elasto-compressive treatment of the lower extremities particularly with elastic stockings. *Der Kassenatzt*, **9**: 1–8.

Stockton L, Flynn M (2009) Sitting and pressure ulcers 1: risk factors, self-repositioning and other interventions. *Nursing Times*, **105**: 12–14.

Stockton L, Gebhardt KS, Clark M (2009) Seating and pressure ulcers: clinical practice guideline. *Journal of Tissue Viability*, **18**: 98–108.

Takahashi M, Black J, Dealey C, Gefen A (2010) Pressure in context. In: *International Review Pressure Ulcer Prevention: Pressure, Shear, Friction and Microclimate in Context A Consensus Document*. London: Wounds International.

Tavakoli K, Rutkowski S, Cope C, Hassall M, Barnett R, Richards M, Vandervord J (1999) Recurrence rates of ischial sores in para- and tetraplegics treated with hamstring flaps: an 8 year study. *British Journal of Plastic Surgery*, **52**: 476–479.

Tennvall GR, Andersson K, Bjellerup M, Hjelmgren J, Oien R (2004) Treatment of venous leg ulcers can be better and cheaper. Annual costs calculation based on an inquiry study. *Lakartidningen*, **101**: 1506–1513.

Theaker C, Mannan M, Ives N, Soni N (2000) Risk factors for pressure sores in the critically ill. *Anaesthesia*, **55**: 221–224.

Top S, Arveschoug AK, Fogh K (2009) Do short-stretch bandages affect distal blood pressure in patients with mixed aetiology leg ulcers? *Journal of Wound Care*, **18**: 439–442.

Vanderwee K, Grypdonck MHF, de Bacquer D, Defloor T (2006) Effectiveness of turning with unequal time intervals on the incidence of pressure ulcer lesions. *Journal of Advanced Nursing*, **57**: 59–68.

Van Gaal BG, Schoonhoven L, Vloet LC, Mintjes JA, Borm GF, Koopmans RT, van Achterberg T (2010) The effect of the SAFE or SORRY? Programme on patient safety knowledge of nurses in hospitals and nursing homes: a cluster randomised trial. *International Journal of Nursing Studies*, **47**: 1117–1125.

van Geffen P, Reenalda J, Veltink PH, Koopman BFJM (2008) Effects of sagittl postural adjustments on seat reaction load. *Journal of Biomechanics*, **41**: 2237–2245.

van Gilder C, MacFarlane GD, Meyer S (2008) Results of nine international pressure ulcer prevalence surveys: 1989–2005. *Ostomy Wound Management*, **54**: 40–54.

van Gilder C, Amlung S, Harrison P, Meyer S (2009) Results of the 2008–2009 international pressure ulcer prevalence survey and a 3-year, acute care, unit-specific analysis. *Ostomy Wound Management*, **55**: 39–45.

van Hecke A, Grypdonck M, Defloor T (2009) A review of why patients with leg ulcers do not adhere to treatment. *Journal of Clinical Nursing*, **18**: 337–349.

Walsh R (2002) Improving diagnosis of malignant leg ulcers in the community. *British Journal of Nursing*, **11**: 604–613.

Waterlow J (1985) A risk assessment card. *Nursing Times*, **81**: 49–55.

Waterlow J (1988) Prevention is cheaper than cure. *Nursing Times*, **84**: 69–70.

World Union of Wound Healing Societies (2008) *Principles of Best Practice: Compression in Venous Leg Ulcers. A Consensus Document*. London: MEP..

Yang D, Morrison BD, Vandongen YK, Singh A, Stacey MC (1996) *Medical Journal of Australia*, **164**: 718–720.

Young T (2004) The 30° tilt position vs the 90° lateral and supine positions in reducing the incidence of non-blanching erythema in a hospital inpatient population: a randomised trial. *Journal of Tissue Viability*, **14**: 88–96.

Zhao G, Hiltabidel E, Liu Y, Chen L, Liao Y (2010) A cross-sectional descriptive study of pressure ulcer prevalence in a teaching hospital in China. *Ostomy Wound Management*, **56**: 38–42.

6 The Management of Patients with Acute Wounds

Introduction

Acute wounds can be defined as wounds of sudden onset and of short duration. They include surgical wounds and traumatic wounds such as burns. Acute wounds can occur in people of all ages and generally heal easily without complication. This chapter considers the specific care needed for patients with acute wounds.

The care of surgical wounds

Surgical wounds are, by their very nature, premeditated wounds. This allows the surgeon to attempt to reduce any risks of complications to a minimum. However, as increasingly sophisticated surgery is performed, often on relatively elderly patients, complications are still a hazard. One aspect of nursing care is to monitor the progress of the wound, so that there is early identification of any problems.

Management of surgical wounds

Patient assessment

This is essential to identify any factors that might affect healing. This topic is covered in more detail in Chapter 2.

Wound assessment

This should identify the method of closure, note the use of any drains and observe for any indication of complications. Westaby (1985) described the main aim of surgical wound closure as being the restoration of function and physical integrity with the minimum of deformity and without infection. The method of wound closure is selected in order to achieve this aim and it

The Care of Wounds: A Guide for Nurses, Fourth Edition. Carol Dealey.
© 2012 Carol Dealey. Published 2012 by John Wiley & Sons, Ltd.

will vary according to the surgery performed. There are three methods of closure: primary closure, delayed primary closure and healing by second intention.

Primary closure

Hippocrates (460–377 BC) was the first to describe this method of wound closure. He called it healing by first intention. The skin edges are held in approximation by sutures, clips, staples or tape. In these wounds the skin edges seal very quickly, first with fibrin from clot formation and then as epithelialisation occurs. Within 48 hours the wound should be totally sealed, thus preventing the ingress of bacteria.

Nursing care
The care of wounds healing by first intention is generally straightforward. A simple island dressing is commonly used to cover the wound at the end of the operation. Several studies have shown that the dressing can be removed after 24–48 hours and need not be replaced, (Cruse and Foord, 1980; Weiss, 1983; Chrintz *et al.*, 1989). Heal *et al.* (2006) undertook a randomised controlled trial comparing removing the dressing after 12 hours followed by normal bathing with leaving the dressing in place for 48 hours in 870 patients who had had minor skin excision. They found no difference in infection rates between the two groups. This study was undertaken in tropical Australia and the results may have been different in a more temperate climate, but they are certainly of interest and worthy of further research.

Some surgeons prefer to cover the wound with a film dressing and leave it in place until the sutures are removed. In addition, some patients seem to prefer to have their wound covered. There have also been several small studies that have compared hydrocolloid, hydroactive and film dressings with simple island dressings (Wikblad & Anderson, 1995; Allen, 1996; Holm *et al.*, 1998). The largest study compared three dressings used on sternotomy wounds: an island dressing, a film dressing and a thin hydrocolloid dressing (Wynne *et al.*, 2004). A total of 737 patients were randomised to one of the three dressings. They found no difference in the incidence of wound infection or healing rates. The island dressing was seen to be the most comfortable and cost-effective of the three dressings. It seems reasonable to conclude that although there may not be a need for a dressing over a surgical incision to prevent infection, use of a dressing is more comfortable for the patient. A simple island dressing appears to be comfortable to wear and remove as well as being relatively cheap.

Surgical wounds should be monitored daily for any indication of complications. Removal of sutures or other types of wound closure is usually carried out under medical supervision.

Delayed primary closure

This method of closure is used when there has been considerable bacterial contamination. Initially, any body cavity is closed and the remaining tissue layers are left open to allow free drainage of pus. After about 5 days, these layers are closed and the wound will heal as any primarily closed wound. Wound drains may be used to assist in the removal of any fluid remaining at the wound base. Two studies (Duttaroy *et al.*, 2009; Cohn *et al.*, 2001) have demonstrated that delayed primary closure was an effective method of treatment for dirty abdominal surgical wounds compared with primary closure. There was a significantly higher incidence of infection in the primary closure group compared with the delayed primary closure group in both studies. Duttaroy *et al.* (2009) also found significantly faster healing and shorter length of stay in the delayed primary closure group.

Nursing care

The aim of management of these wounds is to allow free drainage of any pus. This may be achieved by loose packing of the cavity. As the wound will be sutured at about day 5, the promotion of granulation is not a major aim. If ribbon gauze is used, it should be kept moist and changed regularly to prevent it drying out and adhering to the wound. Alginate rope may also be used, as it is very absorbent and can be removed without pain to the patient. Once the wound is sutured it should be treated as a wound healing by first intention.

Healing by second intention

Healing by second intention describes a wound that is left open and heals by granulation, contraction and epithelialisation. This method may be used for a variety of reasons:

- there may be considerable tissue loss, e.g. radical vulvectomy;
- the surgical incision is shallow, but has a large surface area, e.g. donor sites;
- there may have been infection, for example a ruptured appendix or an abscess may have been drained, and free drainage of any pus is essential.

Nursing care

The care of varying types of surgical wounds will be described here.

Surgical cavities: surgical cavities are generally clean wounds with a healthy bed that would be expected to heal without complication. Harding (1990) suggests that surgical cavities should be boat-shaped in order to heal rapidly without premature surface healing. Simple wound measurement is usually sufficient to monitor healing rates (see Chapter 3). These wounds should also be observed for indications of infection.

Selection of a suitable dressing depends on the position of the wound and the amount of exudate. Vermeulen *et al.* (2010) undertook a systematic review of dressings and topical agents used to manage surgical wounds healing by secondary intention. They concluded that the studies were too small to provide guidance on the treatment of choice. However, they found that foam had been most frequently studied as an alternative to gauze and that it seemed to be preferable in respect of pain reduction, patient satisfaction and nursing time. Alginate packing has also been found to be a useful dressing for this type of cavity wound, although the evidence is limited (Murphy, 2006). Further large studies are required to provide clear evidence as to the most effective treatment regimes.

Skin grafts: skin grafts are widely used in reconstructive surgery following trauma or burns. They may also be used to repair chronic wounds such as pressure sores or leg ulcers. Skin grafting is a technique that permits the transfer of a portion of skin from one part of the body to another. There are several ways of classifying skin grafts. They can be divided into:

(1) autografts – a graft of the patient's own skin;
(2) allografts – a graft taken from another individual;
(3) xenografts – a graft taken from another species.

Grafts can be described according to their thickness. This depends on the amount of dermis that is included in the graft. A full-thickness graft includes the epidermis and all the dermis. A partial or split-thickness graft includes the epidermis and some dermis. This type of graft can be cut to varying thickness depending on need. The graft can also be meshed in order to cover a larger surface area.

Other types of graft are flaps or pedicle grafts, pinch grafts and tissue cultures. Flaps may include other tissue besides skin and one part of the graft is still attached to the original site. This provides a blood supply to the graft until a new blood supply has been established. It is particularly useful in areas where the blood supply is poor and for areas of the face. An example is a gluteal rotation flap to cover the cavity of an ischial pressure sore.

Pinch grafts are small pieces of skin that have been obtained by pinching the area with forceps or lifting with a needle and slicing off with a knife. They have been used as a method of treating leg ulcers, but there is limited evidence as to their success in long-term healing of leg ulcers.

Tissue culture has been developed primarily in burns units, where repeated grafting from the same donor site may be necessary for patients with large surface area burns. A small sample of skin about 2 cm in diameter can be used to culture epithelial sheets many times this size. One of the early studies using this method was carried out by Gallico *et al.* (1984) on two children who had burn injuries affecting more than 95% of their body surface area. Tissue culture provided effective grafts for more than 50% of the body surface. When such extensive burns occur, autografting is very limited because of the lack of appropriate donor sites. Allografting is also used, but they do not always take. Tissue culture can reduce the need for frequent surgery to take further grafts.

Grafts may be sutured or stapled in position or just laid in place. The graft may be left exposed or covered with a dressing to help anchor it in place. The graft must be observed carefully for any indication of infection, oedema or haematoma. It may also be necessary to immobilise the area so that the graft does not slip out of position. Tension over the graft must also be avoided as it may damage the vulnerable blood supply.

Gauze dressings and paraffin gauze have been used to cover grafts, but there is no evidence to determine their effectiveness. Davey *et al.* (2003) described the use of Hyperfix™ in a paediatric burns unit over a 15-year period. It was used for over 700 grafts and found to be an effective covering with only 18 patients (2%) requiring repeat grafts. Peanut oil was routinely applied to the strapping 2 hours before dressing change in order to facilitate its removal without damage to the graft.

Bolster dressings have also been used to assist in securing full-thickness skin grafts to the new site. The purpose of the dressing is to prevent any movement, minimise dead space and reduce seroma or haematoma formation. Traditionally the bolster dressing has been made from paraffin gauze dressings, sometimes wrapped around antiseptic-soaked cotton wool, and tied in place with sutures. There are case reports describing the successful use of silicone net rather than traditional methods (Roh *et al.*, 2008) and a randomised study comparing foam stents with traditional methods (Atherton *et al.*, 2008). There was no significant difference in the level of graft-take between the two groups, but dressing removal was more comfortable.

A small study investigated the use of topical negative pressure therapy (TNP) as a fixative for split-thickness skin grafts (Moisidis *et al.*, 2004). Twenty-two patients were recruited and the donor sites divided into two halves and then each half randomised to either TNP or standard treatment of silicone net, proflavine wool and foam sponge. A narrow bridge of several layers of hydrocolloid separated the two treatments. They found that there was no significant difference in graft take between the two treatments, but quality of the graft-take was significantly better in the TNP group. However, this is a very small study and a larger study is required to determine a definitive outcome.

As the graft becomes vascularised it becomes approximately the same colour as the donor site. In Caucasians, the ideal colour is pink. It is more difficult to assess the vascularity of a graft in darker skins. Coull and Wylie (1990) suggest the use of a colour code along with an assessment chart to monitor the progress of skin flaps. Once a graft has taken it still needs to be handled very carefully as the tissues are still fragile. It should be protected against any extremes of temperature and sunlight. Once the graft is healed the skin should be massaged twice daily with a bland moisturising cream. This helps to improve the suppleness of the skin, as it is likely to be less well lubricated than normal.

A graft may fail to take for a variety of reasons. If there is an inadequate blood supply to the graft bed the microcirculation will fail to grow into the graft and it will necrose from lack of oxygen. Equally, haematoma formation will cause separation of the graft. If the graft slides out of position it will cause separation of some or all of the graft and lead to failure.

Infection, especially from *pseudomonas aeruginosa* and beta haemolytic streptococcus, will also cause failure. Infection will cause pain, odour, itching and redness around the edges of the graft and a low-grade fever (Francis, 1998). It is most likely to occur between the second and fourth post-operative day.

Donor sites: ideally, donor sites are taken from a part of the body where the skin provides a good match for the recipient site. The colour, texture and hair-bearing properties of the skin have to be considered. One of the commonest areas for a donor site is the thigh, where a large area of skin can be obtained.

Donor sites are often described as being more painful than the skin graft for which the removed skin has been used. This is probably, in part, because of the large number of exposed nerve endings. Initially, a donor site is a raw haemorrhagic area. Pressure is needed to stop the bleeding and the wound should be checked regularly in the immediate post-operative period. Analgesia is also necessary and may be needed for several days.

In the past, donor sites have been dressed with paraffin gauze, covered with ordinary gauze, wrapped in wool roll or gamgee and held in place with bandages (Wilkinson, 1997). However, two surveys of plastic surgeons, one in Australia and New Zealand (Lyall & Sinclair, 2000) and one in the UK (Geary & Tiernan, 2009) have shown that alginates were by far the most widely used dressings. Paraffin gauze was only still used by a very small number of surgeons. In the light of this, Geary and Tiernan (2009) suggest that an alginate dressing should be regarded as the standard treatment against which new dressings should be measured.

A systematic review by Wiechula (2003) examined the use of dressings for the management of donor sites. In the analysis the outcomes of using all types of moist wound and non-moist products were compared using meta-analysis. It showed a significant benefit of moist wound products such as films, foams and hydrocolloids compared with non-moist dressings such as paraffin gauze in terms of healing, pain and wound infection. The author also compared different types of products with paraffin gauze. Hydro-colloids were significantly better in terms of healing, pain and wound infection. Films also outperformed paraffin gauze in terms of healing, pain and wound infection. There were insufficient studies of good quality to determine the relative effectiveness of alginates.

A systematic review by Voineskos *et al.* (2009) grouped dressing types into either moist or non-moist categories in order to determine which group of dressings was associated with the least pain, the lowest infection rate and fastest healing rate. The reviewers concluded that many of the studies were of poor quality and that there is no clear evidence of the superiority of moist dressings over non-moist ones and a state of equipoise exists. They did, however, find that moist dressings are less painful than dry ones.

Once the donor site has healed the skin should be kept supple. The use of emollients may be of assistance and should be applied two or three times a day. The patient should be advised to avoid extremes of temperature. If it is not possible to avoid exposing the site to sunlight, sun blockers should be used to cover the area. Donor sites remain susceptible to sunburn for up to a year after healing (Fowler & Dempsey, 1998). A tubular bandage may be applied to donor sites on a lower limb to provide support and to prevent hypertrophy of the scar.

Wound drains: these are inserted to provide a channel to the body surface for fluid that might otherwise collect in the wound. The fluid may be blood, pus, serous exudate, bile or other body fluids. Open drains that drain into the dressing are used very occasionally, but the majority of drains currently used are closed drains.

Closed drains consist of the drain, connection tubing and the collecting receptacle. They usually provide a vacuum and so have a suction effect. Chest drains are closed drains that work rather differently. The purpose of this type of system is to allow air to escape from the chest cavity and bubble into the water in the container. Closed drains are usually inserted through a stab wound adjacent to the incision.

Drains have been used to prevent the collection of fluid in the tissues beneath the wound. However, recent systematic reviews looking at the use of wound drains in a variety of surgical procedures have questioned their value. Systematic reviews of the use of drains after both uncomplicated laproscopic cholecystectomy and uncomplicated open cholecystectomy both found a significant increase in infection rates in those with drains (Gurusamy *et al.*, 2009; Gurusamy & Samraj, 2009). A systematic review of the use of drains for caesarean section found no difference in infection rates between the two groups (Gates & Anderson, 2010) and similar results were found in a review of drains following thyroidectomy (Samraj & Gurusamy, 2008). Two randomised trials, one of breast reduction and the other of laparotomies also found no difference in infection rates between drain and no drain groups (Corion *et al.*, 2009; Baier *et al.*, 2010).

A systematic review of the use of drains in orthopaedic surgery found no difference in infections rates between those with drains and those without. But they did find that those without drains required more reinforcement of their dressings and suffered a higher occurrence of bruising (Parker *et al.*, 2008). Bruising can cause considerable discomfort to patients following hip or knee replacement, so this is an important issue to consider.

It seems reasonable to conclude that with improving surgical techniques and materials, drains do not need to be used as frequently as they have been in the past. However, they are still of some benefit in some types of orthopaedic surgery and when there has been excessive bleeding during surgery.

Managing complications

A variety of complications may occur following surgery. Only those related to the wound will be discussed here.

Haemorrhage

Haemorrhage may occur during surgery, in the immediate post-operative period and up to 10 days afterwards. This is sometimes referred to as primary, intermediary and secondary haemorrhage. The main cause of both primary and intermediary haemorrhage is poor surgical technique. This is either due to failure to control bleeding during surgery or poorly tied blood vessels. As the blood pressure returns to normal levels the clots and ties get pushed off the end of the blood vessel(s) resulting in bleeding. Secondary haemorrhage is invariably associated with infection.

The bleeding may be brisk and rapidly seen, or more insidious. Blood may be seen on the wound dressing or it may drain into a drainage bag. If the bleeding is internal, signs of shock may be the first indication of its presence. If there is only a little bleeding, the blood may ooze into the superficial tissues and show as bruising around the suture line. Slow seeping of blood may lead to haematoma formation when the blood collects in a 'dead space' around the operative site and then clots.

If there is heavy bleeding, further surgery may be needed to find and control the bleeding point. In many cases the bleeding is monitored closely to see if further clotting will resolve the problem. When a haematoma forms it is a potential breeding ground for bacteria. It is sometimes possible to remove a suture in order to evacuate the haematoma.

Infection

Despite considerable improvement in standards of asepsis, post-surgical wound infection still occurs. A review by Leaper *et al.* (2004) estimated that the rate of surgical site infection (SSI) in Europe ranges from 1.5 to 20%, costing an estimated €1.47–19.1 billion. However, the authors concluded that their figures were likely to be an underestimate because of limitations in reporting. Measuring SSI rates is one method used in evaluating standards of care for surgical audit. Although this seems straightforward, it is complicated by a lack of agreement on a definition of SSI. There are three definitions commonly used.

Table 6.1   **US Centre for Disease Control surgical site infection definitions**

	Superficial incisional infection	**Deep incisional infection**	**Organ/space infection**
Time	Within 30 days of surgery	Within 30 days of surgery or 1 year if implant in place	Within 30 days of surgery or 1 year if implant in place
Site	Involves only skin and subcutaneous tissue	Involves deep soft tissues at surgical site	Involves any part of body opened or manipulated during operation
Must have at least one of:	• Purulent drainage from incision • Organisms isolated from incision • Pain, tenderness, swelling, redness or heat around incision AND incision deliberately opened by surgeon (unless negative culture) • Diagnosis by medical doctor	• Purulent drainage from deep incision • Spontaneous dehiscence or deliberate opening of incision following fever or pain (unless negative culture) • Abscess involving deep incision • Diagnosis by medical doctor	• Purulent drainage from a stab wound into the organ/space • Organisms isolated from organ/space • Abscess involving the organ/space • Diagnosis by a medical doctor

- The US Centre for Disease Control (CDC) definition as shown in Table 6.1. This is most widely used, but it is considered to be unreliable (Allami *et al.*, 2005).
- The UK Nosocomial Infection National Surveillance Scheme (NINSS), which is based on the CDC definition, but has two modifications to improve objectivity: pus cells must be present for a positive wound culture; surgeon's diagnosis of infection is excluded. However, the reproducibility of NINSS is low (Wilson *et al.*, 2002).
- A quantitative wound scoring method called ASEPSIS (Wilson *et al.*, 1990). The ASEPSIS wound scoring system, with the grading for the severity of infection, is shown in Figure 6.1. It is more complicated than the other two systems and so is more time-consuming and costly to use.

Ashby *et al.* (2010) undertook a prospective surveillance programme of 7299 trauma and elective orthopaedic patients in one teaching hospital over an 8-year period. Patients' wounds were reviewed on days 2–3 and 4–5 post surgery and a self-assessment form was given to patients to take home and return 2 months later. Sufficient data was collected to be able to assess the wounds using CDC, NINSS and ASEPSIS. They found infection rates of 15.45% (CDC), 11.32% (NINSS) and 8.79% (ASEPSIS), demonstrating the need for a single reproducible definition of SSI if it is to be used as a performance indicator. The authors also discuss the importance of only comparing results where hospitals are using the same standards for data collection (Ashby *et al.*, 2010).

TABLE A

Wound characteristic	Proportion of wound affected (%)					
	0	<20	20–29	40–59	60–79	>80
Serous exudate	0	1	2	3	4	5
Erythema	0	1	2	3	4	5
Purulent exudate	0	2	4	6	8	10
Separation of deep tissues	0	2	4	6	8	10

TABLE B

Criteria for allocation of additional points to ASEPSIS Score

Criterion	Points
Additional treatment	
Antibiotics	10
Drainage of pus under local anaesthetic	5
Debridement of wound (general anaesthetic)	10
Serous discharge	Daily 0–5
Erythema	Daily 0–5
Purulent drainage	Daily 0–10
Separation of deep tissues	Daily 0–10
Isolation of bacteria	10
Stay as inpatient prolonged over 14 days	5

Score **Table A** daily for first week, add points from **Table B** for any criteria satisfied in first 2 months after surgery.

Category of infection: total score 0–10 = satisfactory healing, 11–20 = disturbance of healing; 21–30 = minor wound infection; 31–40 = moderate wound infection; >40 = major wound infection.

Figure 6.1   **The ASEPSIS wound score (from: Wilson, APR, Weavill C, Burridge J, Kelsey MC (1990). Reproduced with kind permission of Elsevier. © 1990, Elsevier)**

As patients have a much shorter hospital stay than in the past, it is important that surveillance should continue after discharge. A study by Jonkers *et al.* (2003) followed patients undergoing cardiac surgery for 90 days. They divided infections into sternal wound infections (SWI) and donor site infections (DSI). They found that considerably more infections were diagnosed at 30 days compared with those identified during hospital admission: SWI rose from 4.7% to 6.8% at 30 days and DSI rose from 1.5% to 4.6% during the same period. They had risen further by 90 days to 9% (SWI) and 7.3% (DSI). They concluded that accurate surveillance should include follow-up after discharge.

It is extremely costly to have surveillance team visiting patients post discharge from hospital and so other means need to be considered. Knaust *et al.* (2009) developed a patient questionnaire based on the CDC to send to patients 10 days following discharge from hospital. Statistical analysis was used to identify the predictive power of each item in the questionnaire. A total of 174 questionnaires were analysed and 3 items were identified as having adequate predictive power: pain, swelling and diagnosis of SSI by a physician. The authors suggest that when SSI is suspected, a follow-up telephone call to ask if the patient was prescribed antibiotics will confirm the diagnosis of SSI and reduce the risk of over-reporting (Knaust *et al.*, 2009).

When measuring the incidence of surgical wound infections it is essential to understand the potential causes. Probably the most important factor to consider is surgical technique. A survey of 117 private sector hospitals in the USA found higher rates of SSI in hospitals that had higher trainee-to-bed ratios and where operations of low complexity were of longer duration (Campbell *et al.*, 2008). Vilar-Compte *et al.* (2009) undertook a 5-year surveillance programme of SSI in patients undergoing breast cancer surgery. They found that the presence of haematoma and length of surgery to be factors associated with SSI. Haematoma is associated with poor surgical technique as it can imply failure to achieve adequate haemostasis and possibly a lack of care in handling the tissues. In this study it would seem that the length of time of operations was associated with more extensive surgery rather than teaching trainees.

Harrington *et al.* (2004) collected prospective data on 4474 patients undergoing cardiac surgery. They identified a number of potential risk factors for SSI and used multivariable analysis to determine which were independent predictors of SSI. They found that obesity, diabetes mellitus and age were all independent risk factors.

Prevention of infection is the responsibility of all the members of the healthcare team and starts pre-operatively. Some surgeons have required that patients bathe or shower using skin antiseptics just before their operation. A systematic review by Webster and Osborne (2011) considered seven trials with a total of 10,157 participants and concluded that there was no clear evidence of any reduction in SSI when using skin antiseptics. There is however, good evidence of the association of SSI with pre-operative hair removal by shaving. Tanner *et al.* (2008) undertook a systematic review of routine pre-operative hair removal and found that there was no difference in SSI rates in those who had hair removal and those who did not. For those operations where hair removal was necessary they found that the use of depilatory creams or hair clipping resulted in a significantly lower incidence of SSI compared with shaving.

The commonest bacteria to cause SSI was found to be *Staphylococcus aureus* in a survey of 251 hospital in England in 2008 and of these infections 59% were methicillin-resistant *Staphylococcus aureus* (MRSA, Health Protection Agency, 2009). A study by Bode *et al.* (2010) showed that the use of pre-operative nasal swabs to identify nasal carriers of *Staphylococcus aureus* and the subsequent treatment of those positive with mupirocin nasal ointment and chlorhexidine soap significantly reduced the incidence of SSI. However, it is not appropriate to use such nasal decontamination routinely (NICE, 2008).

Nursing care
Early identification of signs of infection is important (see also Chapter 3).

Dehiscence

Dehiscence means the breaking down, or splitting open, of all or part of a wound healing by first intention. Complete dehiscence may involve evisceration of the gut, a condition that is commonly known as 'burst abdomen'. If the skin remains intact when the muscle and fascia layers break down, an incisional hernia occurs. It may not become obvious for some months following surgery.

Dehiscence can occur because of systemic and local factors, but will vary according to the type of surgery. One example is obesity, which is a risk factor for SSI and dehiscence in abdominal and thoracic surgery (Molina *et al.*, 2004). In a study of 3158 patients undergoing coronary artery bypass grafts, the incidence of dehiscence was measured in obese patients and non-obese patients. The research team found a significantly higher incidence in the obese group and the greater the obesity, the higher the incidence of dehiscence (Molina *et al.*, 2004). Interestingly, 96% of those with dehiscence also had an SSI.

Improvements in suturing technique and suture materials have reduced the overall incidence of dehiscence. Molina and colleagues (2004) introduced a method of sternal closure for obese patients that reduced the incidence of dehiscence. A study by Shetty *et al.* (2004) compared skin staples with subcuticular vicryl sutures in 110 patients having hip surgery in a randomised study. They found a significantly higher incidence of wound breakdown and infection in those having skin closure using clips.

Nursing care
If a surgical wound starts to break down, the potential cause(s) should be identified and rectified where possible. The wound should be carefully assessed for indications of infection. If major dehiscence, such as a burst abdomen, occurs, the wound will require resuturing. Most wounds are treated conservatively and allowed to heal by granulation and contraction. This is particularly so when infection is present as all purulent material should be allowed free drainage. When this is associated with complete dehiscence of a suture line with some necrosis, as can be seen in Figure 6.2, TNP therapy may be effective in removing the wound debris and preparing the wound for late resuturing.

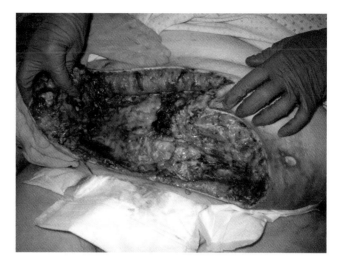

Figure 6.2   **An example of a dehiscent wound with complete breakdown of the suture line**

The wounds may be necrotic or sloughy with a heavy exudate. Management of these types of wounds has been discussed in Chapter 3. If there is only a partial dehiscence of the suture line with little exudate and necrosis then an amorphous hydrogel is appropriate. An alginate or hydrofibre is more appropriate in the presence of heavy exudate or greater dehiscence of the suture line. These dressings cause far less trauma than using traditional methods such as ribbon gauze. Once any cavity is filled with granulation tissue and there is no indication of lingering infection, foam cavity fillers may also be used.

In a few instances the exudate may be excessive and not controlled by dressings. In this situation it may be helpful to consult a colorectal nurse specialist. She/he may suggest that an appliance similar to a drainage bag be used. It has an adhesive backing that can be cut to fit over the wound, while protecting the surrounding skin. The front of the appliance has a hinged lid that allows access to the wound and saves frequent removal. There is usually a tap that allows drainage. The amount of exudate can be measured accurately, which is important for fluid balance. Good wound management of a wound following dehiscence should promote healing and permit the patient to be discharged home for care in the community.

Sinus formation

A sinus is a track to the body surface from an abscess or some material that is an irritant and becomes a focus for infection. A common irritant is suture material. A small case series looked at five patients following spinal surgery who had persistent wound pain at a year post surgery that broke down into a discharging sinus. Investigations identified implant infection and once the implants were removed the pain resolved and the sinuses healed (Gaine *et al.*, 2001). Sinuses can become chronic if the causative factor is not resolved. A sinogram can show the extent of a sinus and help to identify the root problem. Surgical excision or laying open of the sinus is usually the most effective form of management. Once the focus for infection has been removed and free drainage can occur the remaining cavity will heal by granulation and contraction.

Although wide excision is the most appropriate method of managing a sinus, it is not always possible. If the sinus is very deep the opening may be fairly narrow in relation to the sinus size. Irrigation with saline can help to prevent the accumulation of pus and exudate. The easiest dressing to apply is a hydrogel as it can easily be inserted into the sinus via the applicator. It is, therefore, advisable to use a protective skin wipe to protect the skin if there is heavy exudate as the surrounding skin may become macerated.

Fistula formation

A fistula is an abnormal track connecting one viscus with another viscus or a viscus with the body surface. They may develop spontaneously or following surgery. Common examples are: rectovaginal – connecting the rectum and vagina; biliary – allowing leakage of bile to the surface following surgery on the gall bladder and/or bile ducts; faecal – allowing leakage of faecal fluid through the wound, often associated with infection. Persistent leakage of fluid indicates the possible presence of a fistula. Examination of the fluid will usually provide information to indicate the source of the fistula. Any associated infection must also be treated.

Nursing care
The management of fistulae involves care of the surrounding skin, containing and measuring the output and nutritional support. The skin can be protected by the use of ostomy pastes and protective skin wafers. Drainage bags can be applied to collect the output from the fistula. The colorectal nurse specialist may have the greatest skill in applying a suitable drainage bag over the fistula and protecting the skin.

Once the output from the fistula is contained it can be accurately measured. This enables the correct amount of fluid to be given to replace what has been lost. Output may be considerable, sometimes a litre per day. In hospitals where there is a nutrition team they should also be involved in the care of these patients. When it is possible, enteral feeding should be given. If the fistula is high in the gastrointestinal tract then it will be necessary to give parenteral nutrition.

Nienhuijs *et al.* (2003) report on the management and outcomes for 17 patients with entercutaneous fistulae. They followed the treatment described above until spontaneous healing, but 10 patients had skin erosion and required frequent dressing changes. Consequently TNP was applied to these wounds. Patients were given TNP for a median of 25 days (range 14–161 days). Four patients went on to heal spontaneously after a median of 73 days, five patients had surgery to correct the fistula and one patient died, due to extensive metastasis. The four patients who healed spontaneously were discharged home with TNP therapy. Despite the high costs of using TNP, the authors calculated that the cost was cheaper than conventional treatment (€290,394 *v.* €428,311). They noted that as these figures were calculated retrospectively, they should be treated with caution. Undoubtedly the patients in the study were very satisfied with the use of TNP and preferred it to the conventional treatment that they had been given previously.

Evaluation

Regular monitoring of surgical wounds is essential in order to identify any potential complications as early intervention may prevent further problems. Therefore good documentation is essential.

Traumatic wounds

Traumatic injuries can range from a simple cut to a major crushing injury. Major traumatic injury is beyond the remit of this book. It requires surgical intervention and specialised nursing care. Most nurses will be required to care for minor traumatic wounds from time to time. Their care will be considered here.

Minor traumatic wounds

Assessment

Initial assessment should be to identify any life-threatening problems such as airway obstruction, haemorrhage or shock. Vital signs should be recorded. Any of these problems should be addressed before treating the wound. If possible, a history should be obtained of when, where and how the injury occurred. A medical history can highlight any factors that may affect healing of the wound. This information may affect the type of treatment prescribed to manage the wound.

The wound should be assessed for any bleeding. Haemorrhage may be resolved by pressure or require surgical intervention. The presence of any foreign bodies should be noted and the extent and severity of the injury. Khan and Naqvi (2006) suggest that the aim of cleansing traumatic wounds is to remove all organic and inorganic debris and create an environment that will promote wound healing. In addition, cleansing of the wound may be necessary before a full assessment can be made. Loose particles may easily be washed off, but other debris may be more difficult to remove. Bianchi (2000) suggested that pain assessment and management was essential prior to the procedure, especially for children.

Whaley (2004) reviewed the use of potable tap water or normal saline for cleansing traumatic wounds and concluded that the use of tap water did not result in a clinically significant increase in the risk of wound infection when compared with normal saline. However, it must be noted that the studies she reviewed generally lacked power and were of poor quality. A subsequent review by Khan and Naqvi (2006) focusing on antiseptics found that there is still insufficient evidence to determine the best methods of cleansing and cleansers to use. Some A&E departments use cling film to cover a wound until seen by the doctor. This has the advantage of keeping the wound warm and moist and allowing easy observation.

Nursing intervention

Medical assessment and prescription may be necessary before the wound can be dressed. While many nurses are competent to dress minor injuries the following guidelines should be considered.

Patients should be examined by a doctor if:

- the nature and extent of the injury is uncertain;
- there is persistent bleeding;
- suturing is required;
- a foreign body is present;
- tetanus prophylaxis may be necessary;
- the injury occurred to a hospital patient;
- the nurse is uncertain of the appropriate management;
- it is required by nursing policies.

Prior to dressing, the wound should be thoroughly cleaned using saline. Any loose devitalised tissue should be removed. In some instances it may be necessary to shave the area around the wound, if there are hairs that may interfere with the healing process. An appropriate dressing can then be applied. Tetanus prophylaxis will be required if the patient has not had a complete course of tetanus toxoid or if no booster dose has been given for more than 5 years. Depending on the cause of the wound, the doctor may also prescribe a course of antibiotics.

If the patient is not a patient in hospital, he and/or any carer will require information about the management of the wound. Information should also be given concerning whom to contact if any complication occurs. Potential complications such as fever, swelling around the wound, excessive pain or offensive discharge should be described to the patient. Ideally, this information should also be available in written form so that the patient has it for future reference.

Traumatic injuries occur primarily in young and elderly individuals. While most young people will heal easily, this is not necessarily true for older people. They may need to be admitted to hospital for further care.

The management of specific types of traumatic wounds

Abrasions

An abrasion is a superficial injury where the skin is rubbed or torn and it may be extremely sore. It may occur as a result of falling on a gritty surface. Abrasions should be cleaned carefully to ensure that there are no foreign bodies embedded in the wound. In the case of extensive abrasions a general anaesthetic may be required in order to allow adequate cleansing. Failure to remove all the debris may result in unsightly 'tattooing' (Evans and Jones, 1996).

Selection of a suitable dressing depends on the extent and depth of the injury. These wounds are often very sore. Occlusive dressings have been found to reduce the pain, possibly because they keep the nerve endings from drying out. If the abrasion is superficial a film dressing or a thin hydrocolloid or silicone dressing can be applied. Deeper wounds, with a heavier exudate, can be treated with hydrocolloids, silicones, foams or alginates.

Lacerations

A laceration is a wound that penetrates the skin and has a torn and jagged edge. They can be caused by blunt injury that produces shear forces or by a sharp object such as glass (Singer *et al.*, 1997). The aim of treatment is to achieve uncomplicated healing with a functional and cosmetically acceptable scar.

It is important to remove all debris from the wound and any devitalised tissue. This procedure is sometimes called surgical toilet. The best way to manage these wounds is to bring the skin edges together to heal by first intention. This may be achieved by the use of sutures, adhesive strips or tissue adhesive. The choice of material depends on the position of the wound, its extent and the condition of the damaged skin. Suturing is recommended around joints or on the hand where movement is involved. Farion *et al.* (2009) reviewed the use of tissue adhesives for traumatic lacerations in both children and adults. They found no difference in cosmesis between adhesives and standard closures, but tissue adhesives could be applied more quickly and were less painful to use. The authors of the review also noted that there was a small but significant increased rate of dehiscence with tissue adhesives compared with standard closure methods.

One of the commonest positions for a laceration is the pretibial laceration. Davis *et al.* (2004) undertook an audit of A&E departments in a large heavily populated region of the UK and found that the mean incidence of estimated patients with pretibial laceration was 5.2/1000 A&E attendances. The extent of the injury can vary and Dunkin *et al.* (2003) has proposed a method of classifying these wounds:

- I – laceration;
- II – laceration or flap with minimal haematoma and/or skin edge necrosis;
- III – laceration or flap with moderate to severe haematoma and/or necrosis;
- IV – major degloving injury;

Dunkin *et al.* (2003) have also provided a useful management algorithm for the management of each type of laceration. Fairly obviously types III and IV require surgical intervention. Type I lacerations should have the skin edges opposed and then held together with short, wide adhesive strips. The wound is covered with a non-adherent dressing and a crepe bandage applied from toe to knee. It may be appropriate to use a wool bandage under the crepe bandage in order to provide additional protection. Patients should be encouraged to mobilise and to elevate their leg when sitting in order to reduce any oedema. Type II is also managed with use of adhesive strips and supportive bandages, after any haematoma has been evacuated, the non-viable wound edges trimmed and the wound edges apposed. Both these type of lacerations should heal without complication. Failure to do so indicates that the injury is more serious than originally recognised (Dunkin *et al.*, 2003).

If there is any risk of infection as a result of severe contamination of the wound at the time of injury, primary closure is not appropriate. Conservative treatment of antibiotics and the use of dressings such as an amorphous hydrogel is preferable. An iodine impregnated low-adherent dressing may also be used for a short period of time. Once the wound is clean, skin grafting is the fastest method of wound closure.

Finger-Tip injuries

Crushing finger-tip injuries are very common in children, mainly caused by fingers being caught in the house or car doors. A 5-year survey of hand injuries in children aged 0–6 years undertaken in Sweden found that finger-tip injuries were the most common (166/455) in children of 1–5 years (Ljungberg *et al.*, 2003). They can also occur in adults as a result of occupational injuries (Yeo *et al.*, 2010). As with any injury, careful assessment is required to determine management. The PNB classification (pulp, nail, bone) has 7–8 subdivisions for each component, which allows very precise description of the injury. Muneuchi *et al.* (2005) used it to determine when surgery was required and found it to be a useful tool. Yeo *et al.* (2010) described the management of the range of finger-tip injuries recognising the importance of retaining maximum function as well as an aesthetic appearance.

The use of adhesive tapes over the finger tip can be an effective way of holding the wound edges together and then protecting the finger by applying a tubular bandage. Collier (1996) suggests that it is important to use dressings that will not adhere to the wound as adherent dressings will cause pain and further trauma at dressing change. Given that many of the patients are children this is an important consideration. Suitable dressings might be hydrocolloids or adhesive foams that can be retained without bulky dressings or strapping.

Freedman *et al.* (2005) undertook a small randomised study of adults with finger-tip injuries not involving flexor tendon insertion, comparing the topical growth factor becaplermin with surgery. They found there was a significantly faster return to work and healing rate, less functional impairment and shorter course of physiotherapy in the growth-factor group, resulting in significantly lower treatment costs. Another small randomised study compared a lipido-colloid dressing with daily gauze dressings and found a significantly faster healing time in the lipido-colloid group (Ma *et al.*, 2006). However, this study was seriously underpowered, limiting the generalisability of the findings.

Mammalian and human bites

Patients presenting with mammalian bites account for 1% of visits to A&E departments (Medeiros and Saconato, 2001) As many as 74% of bites are from dogs, other animals causing problems include cats, rats, squirrels and, occasionally, snakes. As well as animal bites, patients also present with human bites, usually as a result of physical violence such as a punch to the mouth, which results in injury to the knuckles (Higgins *et al.*, 1997).

Dendle (2009) suggested that the main complications are tissue damage from the bite, the risk of infection and psychological distress. In the case of human bites there is also the risk of transmission of diseases such as HIV or hepatitis B from human bites. Higgins *et al.* (1997) stress the importance of not underestimating these wounds. After reviewing the evidence for the use of prophylactic antibiotics after mammalian bites, Medeiros and Saconato (2001) concluded that there was some evidence that it was beneficial after human bites, but not after dog or cat bites. Dendle (2009) suggested that it might be helpful to identify those likely to be at high risk of infection:

- puncture and crush wounds (especially cat bites);
- wounds that penetrate bone, joint, tendons, vascular structures;
- wounds on the hands, feet, face or genitalia;
- delayed presentation greater than 8 hours;
- patients who are immunocompromised or who have oedematous conditions.

Careful cleansing is essential in order to assess the extent of the injury. Saline or an antimicrobial such as povidone iodine should be used. Surgical debridement or exploration may be necessary to remove devitalised tissue, skin tags or any foreign bodies. Large cuts and facial wounds need suturing. Delayed primary closure may be used for some wounds. Chen *et al.* (2000) monitored that outcome for 145 mammalian bite wounds that were treated by primary closure. They found there was an infection rate of 5.5% and considered that this was an acceptable risk for wounds where a good cosmetic result was essential. However, they also noted that appropriate selection of patients was important.

Puncture wounds should be left open because of the risk of infection. The wound should be protected. An iodine impregnated low-adherent dressing may be suitable, unless there is a moderate to heavy exudate. Although many bite wounds are managed in the community, hospital referral is essential for those causing severe injuries including involvement of bone, joint, tendon or nerve, where there are signs of systemic infection or cellulitis, where surgery is required, bites with puncture wounds and in immunocompromised patient (Dendle, 2009). Patients with bite wounds should be followed up to ensure that there has been uncomplicated healing and the patient has regained full function of the affected area.

Skin tears

Skin tears are caused either by friction or by a combination of friction and shearing associated with thin, fragile skin. Thomas *et al.* (1999) suggest that up to 1.5 million people living in care institutions in the USA suffer a skin tear each year. A survey of 154 nursing home residents revealed that they occurred mostly on the arms in very elderly people who were frail, had limited mobility, poor appetite and ecchymosis (McGough-Csarny & Kopac, 1998). They can be classified according to severity using a classification system devised by Payne and Martin (1993) and can be seen in Table 6.2.

There is limited evidence to determine the best method for managing skin tears. Sutures are not an option as the skin is too fragile and they would cause further damage. Meuleneire (2002) reported on 88 patients with Category I or II (scant tissue loss) that were managed using a silicone-coated net dressing. The same protocol was followed for all wounds. The flap and wound bed were irrigated and the flap gently returned to as close approximation as possible. The wound was covered with silicone-coated net dressing, a secondary low-adherent dressing applied and then a light compression bandage applied to reduce any oedema. The secondary dressing was changed daily for 3 or 4 days and then daily until day 7 when all dressing layers were removed. The wound was then protected using a low-adherent dressing for a further 4–5 days. A total of 83% of the wounds had healed by day 8. The remaining 17% that did not heal in this

Table 6.2   **Skin tear classification (based on Payne & Martin, 1993)**

Category	Subcategory	Definition
I	Linear type	Epidermis and dermis pulled in one layer from supporting structures resulting in skin tear in a straight line
	Flap type	The epidermis and dermis are separated, but the epidermal flap covers the dermis to within 1 mm of the wound margin
II	Scant loss of tissue	An actual loss of tissue no greater than 25% of flap size
	Large loss of tissue	Loss of tissue where more than 25% of the flap has been lost
III		Entire loss of tissue, either at the time of injury or later following necrosis of the flap

time did not do so because of either bleeding or infection. The infection was a consequence of delay in initial treatment as all the infected wounds were treated 6 hours or more after the injury.

Edwards *et al.* (1998) undertook a pilot study to compare four dressings: a film, a thin hydrocolloid, a foam and a combination of adhesive strips and low-adherent dressing on skin tears (no indication of severity was given). Fifty-four patients were recruited to the study, but 24 cases were withdrawn, 14 of these (12 film dressing and 2 hydrocolloid) because the wound was not progressing or it was infected. Of the 30 that completed the study only 13 had healed by day 7 and a further 12 by day 14 and 5 remained unhealed. The combination dressing performed better than the other dressings as about two-thirds had healed by day 7 and the remainder by day 14. However, these numbers are very small and no real conclusions can be drawn, other than the need for further research.

A best practice statement has recently been published following a review of the evidence (All Wales Tissue Viability Nurse Forum, 2011). The statement basically follows the approach taken by Meuleneire (2002), but suggests leaving the dressing in place for 5 days to encourage the skin flap to adhere to underlying tissues. It is also suggested that the outer-side of the dressing is marked with arrows to indicate the direction of removal so that traction on the flap is minimised. The wound should be carefully monitored for signs of infection.

The burn injury

Burns are traumatic wounds, but because of the specialised care required, they need to be considered separately from other traumatic wounds. Burns are measured in terms of the percentage of total body surface area (TBSA) that is affected and they are divided into complex and non-complex burns.

A European working group have developed guidelines for the management of partial-thickness burns outside of specialist burns centres (Alsbjörn *et al.*, 2007). They have proposed guidance on when patients should be referred a burns centre:

- all full-thickness burns;
- partial-thickness burns involving more than 15% TBSA in adults or 10% in children or the elderly;
- burns of the face, hands, feet, armpits, popliteal region, genitals;
- chemical or electrical burns;
- circumferential burns;
- burns associated with inhalation injuries, trauma or disease;
- suspicion of non-accidental injury

The burn care required by these patients is beyond the remit of this book.

Aetiology

A burn is an injury caused by excessive heat. It primarily damages the skin, causing tissue destruction and coagulation of the blood vessels of the affected area. Burn damage consists of three areas or zones (Hettiaratchy & Dziewulski, 2004a). The central zone is the *zone of coagulation* and at this point there is coagulation of the tissue proteins and thus irreversible damage and tissue loss. The *zone of stasis* surrounds the zone of coagulation and there is decreased tissue perfusion in this zone. However, if tissue perfusion is increased promptly it is possible to prevent the tissue damage extending into this zone. The third and outer zone is the *zone of hyperaemia* and here tissue perfusion is increased. Generally this area will recover unless the burn becomes severely infected or there is prolonged hypoperfusion.

Burns can be divided into four categories depending on their cause.

- *Thermal*: caused by flame, hot water or steam, other hot liquids and hot surfaces. Smoke inhalation injuries may be associated with fire casualties.
- *Chemical*: caused by spillage of strong acids, alkalis or other corrosive substances. These are usually industrial injuries. Damage to vital organs can occur if the chemicals are absorbed into the blood supply.
- *Electrical*: caused by an electrical current passing through the body. The internal damage may be considerably greater than is obvious from the skin appearance. Such burns may also be associated with thermal injury.
- *Radiation*: caused by overexposure to industrial ionising radiation or following radiotherapy treatment. (Reactions to radiotherapy are covered in more detail from page 216.)

Although burn injuries are usually described as accidental, it has been suggested that some individuals are more likely to suffer from them than others (Hettiaratchy & Dziewulski, 2004a).

- *Young children*: 20% of all burn injuries are in young children, predominantly boys. Most of these injuries (61%) are the result of scalds.
- *Children aged 5–14 years*: 10% of burns occur in this group and may be as a result of illicit activity such as playing with fireworks or petrol or misuse of electrical equipment.
- *Adults of working age*: around 60% of burns occur in this group generally as a result of flame injury. About one-third of the burns in this group are because of work-related injury. Similar numbers have been found in developing countries, but these flame injuries are from open fires and paraffin stoves used for cooking (Eyal *et al.*, 2006).
- *Elderly people*: 10% of burns occur in this group, often as a result of infirmity or disability.
- *Additional factors*: within all age groups there other predisposing factors that can increase the risk of burn injury. They include medical conditions such as epilepsy, psychiatric illness, alcoholism and social conditions. A review by Edelman (2007) considered socioeconomic status as a risk factor for burn injury and concluded the following increased the risk of burn injury: poverty, lack of education and unemployment; large and single-parent families; and substandard housing, lack of running water and overcrowding.

Incidence

It is estimated that around 250,000 people suffer burn injury each year in the UK (National Burn Care Review Committee, 2001). Out of this group around 175,000 people attend A&E as a result of their injury and for 13,000 it is sufficiently severe to require admission to hospital. About 1000 people, half of whom are children under 12 years, have such severe burns that they require fluid resuscitation. It should also be noted that globally around 322,000 people die from their burns each year (Enoch *et al.*, 2009).

The figures for burn injury in the UK are similar to those in other developed counties (Hettiaratchy and Dziewulski, 2004b). However, in developing countries it is likely to be much higher, for example, it is thought that 2 million of the 500 million people in India have suffered a burn injury. Mortality rates are also likely to be higher in countries with a high level of poverty. Poor housing, overcrowding and the use of open fires for cooking are likely factors in the high incidence of fires in developing countries.

Staff should be aware of the possibility of non-accidental injury to children. A large American study of 15,802 children aged 12 years or younger found that 5.8% of children admitted to burn centres were suspected of suffering from child abuse-related injuries (Thombs, 2008). James-Ellison *et al.* (2009) undertook a smaller matched cohort study of 145 children under the age of 3 years and found that 2.8% were the result of non-accidental injury. Chester *et al.* (2006) undertook a detailed retrospective study of 440 children under the age of 16 years admitted to a regional burns unit over a 2-year period. Initially, concerns were raised in over 40.5% (178) of the children. However, after further investigation it was determined that 41 (9.3%) were because of neglect by parents and 4 (0.9%) were due to deliberate abuse. The remainder were all accidental. The authors were concerned about the numbers of injuries due to neglect and suggest that this requires more attention. Neglected children were more likely to be from single-parent families, have parents who were drug uses, have delayed presentation and a lack of first aid. Their burns were likely to be deeper and to require skin grafting compared with accidental injuries. Abused children were likely to be younger, have larger burns with inconsistent mechanisms of injury (Chester *et al.*, 2006; Thombs, 2008). Degraw *et al.* (2010) studied 147 children with burns who were referred to 19 abuse consultation teams in the USA during 1 year. They found that 24 (16.3%) of the children also had fractures, supporting the recommendation of the American Association of Paediatrics that all children under 2 years of age and where abuse is suspected should have skeletal surveys performed. The National Institute for Health and Clinical Excellence (NICE, 2009) has provided guidance on when to suspect child maltreatment for all aspects of child care. Most A&E departments will have adapted this into specific processes for staff to follow.

First aid treatment of burns

Everyone should be aware of simple first aid for burns. Box 6.1 summarises the basic guidance. The principle treatment is to remove the injured person from the source of heat and apply cold running water over the affected area for 20 minutes. Lawrence and Wilkins (1986) demonstrated that the sub-cutaneous temperature continues to rise after the burn injury occurs. Thus, if a burn injury at $100\,°C$ lasts for 10 seconds, the affected tissue will take 3 minutes to return to normal body temperature. Application of cold water within 10 seconds of the injury can reduce the 'burn-time' to 30 seconds. Ice or iced water should never be used because of the risk of hypothermia (New South Wales Health, 2008).

Application of cool water to reduce burn damage is only effective within 3 hours of injury, but it can be used to reduce pain on minor burns. A variety of cool pads are sold as first aid kits. Cuttle and Kimble (2010) suggest that they are not as effective as cold running water and may make it more difficult to assess large burns. However, these dressings do appear to reduce pain and so they may be useful for minor burns.

> **Box 6.1 The first aid treatment of burns (based on NHS Choices UK: www.nhs.uk)**
>
> - Stop the burning process as soon as possible, by removing the person from the source of heat or putting out the fire
> - Turn off the electricity in the case of electric burns
> - Remove any clothing or jewellery near the burn area, but do not remove anything stuck to the burnt skin
> - Cool the burn with cool water for 10–30 minutes, ideally within 20 minutes of the injury occurring
> - Do NOT use ice or iced water, creams or greasy substances such as butter
> - Layer cling film over the burn rather than wrapping it round a limb
> - A clear plastic bag can be used over burns on the hand
> - Seek qualified help quickly – especially if the burn is extensive

The severity of injury

The skin is the organ of the body that usually suffers the greatest damage from a burn injury. Depending on the extent of the injury, several layers may be affected. It is common to describe the severity of a burn according to its depth and extent. Burns are divided as follows.

- *Superficial burns* – only the upper strata of the epithelium are damaged. The stratum basale is unaffected.
- *Superficial dermal burns* – these burns extend beyond the epidermis into the top layers of the dermis. They are associated with blistering.
- *Deep dermal burn* – the burn extends into the deeper layers of the dermis and may involve hair follicles or sweat glands.
- *Full-thickness burns* – there is full destruction of the epidermis and dermis. The damage extends into the subcuticular layer and may involve muscle and bone.

The extent of the burn is determined by the measurement of the surface area of the affected part, excluding erythema. This is described in terms of a percentage of the whole body. Various methods of achieving this have been described. An *ad hoc* method is to measure the area using the palm of the hand. The palmar surface of the patient is equal to 1% of the body surface area in adults and 1.5% in children. When making the initial assessment of a burn-injured patient, it is most common to use the 'Rules of Nine', (Wallace, 1951). Figure 6.3 shows how the body is divided into sections, each measuring 9% of the whole, or multiples of 9%. The percentages for each affected area are then totalled. Thus, if one arm and the front of the trunk were affected, this would be described as 27% burns.

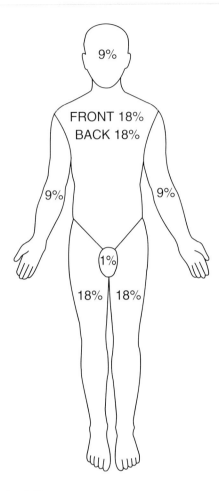

Figure 6.3   **The Rule of Nines**

However, the Rule of Nines may overestimate the extent of the injury. Once the initial emergency treatment has been carried out, a re-assessment of the extent of the injury is usually made. A more accurate picture can be obtained using a Lund and Browder chart (see Figure 6.4). Lund and Browder (1944) developed a system for assessing burn injury that not only divides the body into smaller areas, but also considers the age of the patient. Body proportions alter during childhood, so that the front of the head is 8.5% of the whole in a child of 1 year, but only 4.5% of the whole in a 15-year-old. Patient management may need to be adapted once this re-assessment has been made.

Burn oedema

Almost immediately after injury, oedema starts to collect beneath the damaged tissue. This is typically maximal within 24 hours of the injury,

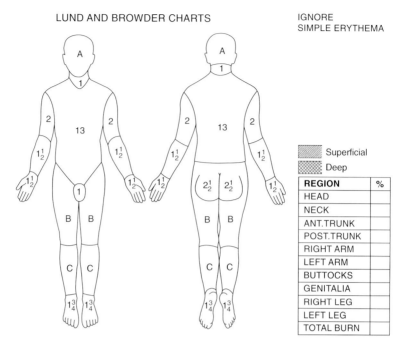

LUND AND BROWDER CHARTS

IGNORE
SIMPLE ERYTHEMA

REGION	%
HEAD	
NECK	
ANT.TRUNK	
POST.TRUNK	
RIGHT ARM	
LEFT ARM	
BUTTOCKS	
GENITALIA	
RIGHT LEG	
LEFT LEG	
TOTAL BURN	

RELATIVE PERCENTAGE OF BODY SURFACE AREA
AFFECTED BY GROWTH

AREA	AGE 0	1	5	10	15	ADULT
A=$\frac{1}{2}$ OF HEAD	$9\frac{1}{2}$	$8\frac{1}{2}$	$6\frac{1}{2}$	$5\frac{1}{2}$	$4\frac{1}{2}$	$3\frac{1}{2}$
B=$\frac{1}{2}$ OF ONE THIGH	$2\frac{3}{4}$	$3\frac{1}{4}$	4	$4\frac{1}{2}$	$4\frac{1}{2}$	$4\frac{3}{4}$
C=$\frac{1}{2}$ OF ONE THIGH	$2\frac{1}{2}$	$2\frac{1}{2}$	$2\frac{3}{4}$	3	$3\frac{1}{4}$	$3\frac{1}{2}$

Figure 6.4   **Lund & Browder chart**

but can last for up to 3 or 4 days. As plasma continues to leak into the tissues, there is a risk of hypovolaemia developing. Without treatment, burns shock can develop and is potentially fatal. If the burn is on the face, neck or chest, the swelling from the oedema may cause obstruction of the airway. Patients with facial burns are admitted for 24 hours as a precaution. Treatment must ensure that the effects of burn oedema are minimised.

The management of burn injuries

When considering the management of burns, the extent of the injury must be defined as the treatment varies drastically between complex and non-complex burns. Non-complex burns may be treated in the out-patient department, but anyone with complex burns must be admitted to hospital.

Complex burns

Depending on the circumstances, it may be necessary to provide initial resuscitation before transferring a patient to a burn care unit. Gordon and Goodwin (1997) describe the importance of the primary assessment of the patient that includes the ABCDEF assessment

- *A = airway,*
- *B = breathing.* Check airway – endotracheal intubation may be needed if there are deep burns to face, neck or mouth or any indication of respiratory distress.
- *C = circulation.* Check pulse – may be absent or show signs of dysrythmias following electric burn.
- *D = disability or neurological deficit.* Identify any associated trauma. Signs of mental confusion or disorientation may be an indication of a pre-existing conditions, hypoxia or unrecognised injury.
- *E = exposure and evaluation.* All jewellery or clothes should be removed from the burn-injured area because of the risk of constriction when burn oedema develops. This also allows for a rapid assessment of the full extent of the injury, using the Rules of Nine. The patient should be kept warm; a space blanket is ideal.
- *F = fluid resuscitation.* Establish an intravenous infusion - this is essential for all burns greater than 15% TBSA in adults and 10% in children. Blood samples may be taken at the same time. Catheterise the bladder if the burns are 25% or more TBSA – urinary output will indicate inadequate rehydration as well as renal function.

Analgesia may also be required, especially for those with superficial burns as they are very painful (Hettiaratchy & Papini, 2004).

It is also important to obtain a full history of the cause of the injury from the patient, a relative or the ambulance crew. This may provide information indicating potential complications such as smoke inhalation. Analgesia, such as inhalational analgesia or systemic analgesia, may be given depending on the condition of the patient.

When the patient's condition has been stabilised by the above measures, urgent transfer to the burn care unit can take place. Once in the care of a burns team a more detailed assessment of the patient and the extent of the burn injury using a Lund and Browder chart is undertaken. Essentially, assessment of the extent of damage is by visual assessment. However, Mileski *et al.* (2003) found that a Doppler flow meter could be a useful tool to measure tissue perfusion, thus allowing easier differentiation between the different zones of the burn injury. They found that serial measurements had a positive predictive value of 81% for identifying non-healing wounds.

Non-Complex burns

Managing minor burns requires assessment of both the patient and the wound as in any other type of wound. Assessment of the patient has been discussed in Chapter 2 and wound assessment and management in Chapter 3. Specific aspects of the care of minor burns are discussed here.

Patient assessment

- *Burn aetiology*: discover the cause of the injury. Non-accidental injury must be considered if the history seems inconsistent with the burn appearance. The risk of infection is always present in the burn-injured patient.
- *Pain*: analgesia may be required for pain.
- Nutrition: nutritional status should be identified. Advice on nutrition may be necessary as there will be increased nutritional demands on the body. Prelack *et al.* (2007) have provided practical guidelines for nutritional support. Although aimed primarily at the management of complex burns, they have relevance for those with less complex injuries.
- *Sleep*: pain or anxiety may affect sleep patterns.
- *Early psychological care*: many patients will be very frightened. It is important to provide re-assurance and explanation to the patient and the family.
- *Later psychological care*: a burn injury can be extremely disfiguring. Body image may be profoundly altered causing distress and loss of self-esteem. Many patients may have fears of disfigurement or disability. Some may fear loss of loved ones as a result of the scarring. Specific fears should be identified and addressed.

Wound assessment

Initial assessment of a burn injury includes the extent and depth of the burn. The use of a Lund and Browder chart has already been described. The zone of hyperaemia should not be included when calculating the burn area. Identifying the depth of a burn is not always easy to do, especially as a burn injury may have varying depths. Table 6.3 shows how it is possible to differentiate between the different wound depths.

A European working party have produced guidelines for managing partial-thickness burns, including a very useful algorithm showing the management pathway (see Figure 6.5, Alsbjörn *et al.* (2007).

Wound management

Superficial burns

Superficial Burns may be very painful and require analgesia. Fowler (2003) suggested treating them like minor sunburn with aloe vera gel or other after-sun lotions. Aloe vera gel is soothing and feels cooling and thus helps to alleviate the pain.

Table 6.3   **Identifying burn wound depth (from Fowler, 2003)**

Depth of burn	Skin structures affected	Indicators
Superficial	Upper strata of epithelium	• Skin intact, red and very painful • Blanches under fingertip pressure • Usually no blisters, but may form in the 48-hour period after injury
Superficial dermal	Epidermis and upper layers of dermis	• Blister form immediately with a pink/red wound bed below • Wound areas may be red and moist and exuding • Easily observable brisk capillary refill • Painful and sensitive to skin changes
Deep dermal	Epidermis down to deep layers of dermis, possibly hair follicles and sweat glands	• Burn creamy/white • May have large blisters • Initially burn has little moisture • Slight pain with insensate areas not sensitive to pin prick
Full thickness	Complete destruction of epidermis and dermis, may involve muscle or tendon	• Burn appears waxy white, cherry red, grey or leathery • Little or no pain – but may be areas on the edges of the burn that are not so deep and therefore painful

Superficial dermal burns

Superficial dermal burns require careful cleansing with warm saline or tap water to remove all loose debris in the first instance. They have traditionally been treated with paraffin gauze dressings or silver sulphadiazine cream and covered with gauze and a bandage. Although healing will occur with this regime, there are several disadvantages. The dressings are bulky and hinder washing around the affected area. They may also be painful to remove, although it may not be necessary to remove the wound contact layer until the wound is healed and it separates spontaneously. An internet survey of burn centres across the world found that silver dressings, especially silver sulphadiazine are still the most widely used dressings (Hermans, 2007). Although there are a number of limitations to the survey the difference in the use of silver in comparison with other dressings was so large as to make it a reasonable conclusion.

Modern products are easier to use and are also more comfortable for patients, especially when being removed. There is limited evidence to determine best practice, but the available evidence seems to favour modern products. Although Alsbjörn *et al.* (2007) did not name specific products because of variations in availability across Europe they proposed the characteristics of a suitable dressing:

- maintains a moist healing environment;
- absorbs excessive wound exudate;

Examine depth and assess area
- Partial thickness burns – wet/painful/red white/pink white
- Full-thickness burn – dry/no pain/grey/white/brownish/looks like normal skin without sensation
- Use Rule of Nines for area
- Use Lund & Browder charts for children

Prepare the wound
- Apply cold water as soon as possible
- Remove clothing, keep patient warm
- Offer pain relief as soon as required
- Tetanus prophylaxis if not current (>5 years)
- Clean and disinfect wound
- Remove loose skin and blisters (>2% TBSA)
- Puncture blisters <2% TBSA

Cover wound with appropriate dressing
- Modern dressings: e.g. hydrocolloids, hydrofibre, silicone, alginate, polyurethane dressings
- Traditional dressings: e.g. silver sulphadiazine

Initial referrals
See list on p. 206

Late referrals
- Not healed in 10–14 days
- Late presentation of pain, fever, exudate, redness, odour, malaise

Very late referrals

Post-wound care
- Moisturise healed wound
- Protect from sunburn for 12 months
- Prevent itching with low-pressure garments, extra moisturisers & oral medications as necessary
- Discuss with patient regarding return to work
- Patient to return if surface changes occur eg blisters or new wounds
- Offer psychological support if necessary

Figure 6.5 **Clinical algorithm for the management of partial-thickness burns (from Alsbjörn B, Gilbert P, Hartmann B, Kaźmierski M, Monstrey S, Palao R, Roberto MA, van Trier A, Voinchet V (2007). Reproduced with kind permission of Elsevier. © 2007, Elsevier). TBSA, total body surface area**

- conforms to the wound position;
- non-adherent but maintains a close contact with the wound;
- easy to apply and remove without causing pain;
- provides a barrier to reduce risk of contamination and infection.

Other dressings that can be used on minor burns include flat foam dressings, silicone net dressings and hydrogels. The foam dressings are comfortable and can be held in place with tape or a tubular net. Hydrogels can give a cooling sensation when applied that may be comforting to the patient. Silicone net dressings are widely used as they can be left in place for 7–14 days and the secondary dressing changed when necessary.

Whatever dressing is used, the patient and wound should be reviewed between 48–72 hours when the local oedema has subsided (Fowler, 2003). This review is especially important for patients who are being managed at home and are attending the outpatient department.

Deep dermal and full-thickness burns
Deep dermal and full-thickness burns generally require early excision of necrotic tissue and skin grafting for speedy healing.

After care

Evaluation of the burn wound involves both monitoring of the wound as it progresses towards healing and of the healed wound. Any non-complex burn that fails to heal within 3 weeks should be referred to a specialist unit.

Once the wound is healed, special care needs to be taken of the newly formed epithelia. The newly healed tissue should be moisturised regularly and sun-block should be used to protect it from further damage from the sun. Alsbjörn *et al*. (2007) recommend that a cream with a sun protection factor of 25 should be used.

Potential problems that can develop are contractures and hypertrophic scarring. If they occur patients should be referred to a burns centre as a late referral for advice and management. A few patients will develop permanent pigmentation changes. This is possibly because of damage to the melanocytes in the basal layer of the epidermis. It can present as either apigmentation or hyperpigmentation. It is not possible to predict when it will occur.

Radiation reactions

Radiation reaction is the reaction of the skin to the effects of radiotherapy and is limited to the treatment field or its exit point. Strictly speaking, a radiation reaction is not a wound. However, the skin reaction is akin to a superficial burn and has the potential for ulceration. There is limited research into the management of what can be a very painful problem.

Aetiology

Ionising radiation or radiotherapy is the mainstay of cancer treatment. Treatment is usually given in a series of doses, ranging from daily to weekly, although a small number of patients will receive just one dose. A course of treatment may last up to 8 weeks. Salvo *et al.* (2010) suggest that up to 90% of patients will have a skin reaction at the treatment site. Radiation reactions are most likely to occur when the treatment field is close to the body surface, such as the head or neck, or if it includes axillae, under breasts, perineum or groin. The reaction is dose-dependent, that is the more frequent the treatment or the higher the dose, the more likely the reaction. A reaction may occur during a course of treatment or after it is completed. Within 6 weeks of completion of treatment, all but the most severe reactions have disappeared.

The classification of radiation reactions

The severity of radiation reactions are generally classified using the grading system developed by the Radiation Therapy Oncology Group (RTOG) (Cox *et al.*, 1995) and recommended by the College of Radiographers in the UK.

(0) No change over baseline.
(1) Follicular, faint or dull erythema.
(2a) Tender or bright erythema with/without dry desquamation.
(2b) Patchy moist desquamation, moderate oedema.
(3) Confluent wet desquamation; pitting oedema.
(4) Ulceration, haemorrhage, necrosis.

In a review of the subject, McQuestion (2006) considered that patients were more vulnerable to radiation reactions if they had comorbidities such as diabetes or renal failure, older age, poor nutritional status, chronic sun exposure, smoking, previous lymphocele aspiration. Those receiving treatment to sites where two surfaces are in contact such as the breast or perineum are particularly vulnerable.

Preventative skin care

Steps can be taken to help reduce the risk of radiation reactions. While the presence of comorbidities cannot be altered, actions such as the avoidance of the use of deodorants or aftershave can help. NHS Quality Improvement Scotland (NHS QIS) (2010) provides useful information in the form of a best practice statement. Box 6.2 provides a summary of the recommended skin care. Unfortunately, despite this guidance, there is considerable variation in practice in relation to the advice given to patients concerning how the skin within the treatment field should be managed while radiotherapy is in progress (Faithfull *et al.*, 2002; Grobler *et al.*, 2010).

Wells and colleagues reviewed the findings of their study of 357 patients undergoing radiotherapy and concluded that level of skin discomfort were

> **Box 6.2 Summary of recommendations for skin care during radio-therapy treatment**
>
> - Wash treatment site daily using mild unperfumed soap
> - Avoid having a very hot shower, especially if the water jets are powerful
> - Pat area dry with soft towel, avoiding friction
> - Do not apply deodorants, perfume or aftershave to the treatment site
> - Apply a mild emollient twice daily, ensuring emollient at room temperature
> - For men having radiotherapy to face or neck – use an electric razor rather than a wet shave
> - If the axilla is part of the treatment site – do not shave during treatment
> - If swimming, wash off chlorinated water as it is drying to skin and apply emollient
> - Wear loose clothing over treatment site to avoid friction
> - Avoid sun exposure where possible and use sunblock if it is unavoidable

lower than they had expected (Wells *et al.*, 2004). They concluded that consistent advice, skin hygiene and regular assessment were major factors in reducing problems. It is interesting to postulate that a reason for previous reports of severe skin problems may have been as a result of the type of advice given some years ago that patients should not wash the treatment area. Happily, that advice is now seen as outdated

Managing radiation reactions

A systematic review of treatments for radiation reactions by Salvo *et al.* (2010) found that there is limited evidence to guide the practitioner, in part because the trials studied a wide variety of products, tended to be small and used a range of outcome measures. NHS QIS (2010) provides guidance for the management of each grade of radiation reaction.

RTOG Score 1 and 2a

The skin should be kept clean and supple with soap and water. A simple moisturiser such as aqueous cream can be soothing applied to the area twice daily. If aqueous cream is not effective an alternative cream may help. There is much anecdotal evidence of the benefits of using aloe vera gel and Heggie *et al.* (2002) undertook a study of 225 patients undergoing treatment for breast cancer comparing aloe vera gel with aqueous cream. They found that aqueous cream was significantly better that aloe vera gel in reducing dry desquamation and pain. However, Wells *et al.* (2004) did not find this to be the case when comparing aqueous cream with either sucralfate cream or no cream. They concluded that patients should be given the choice to use a cream or not. If there is itching on the site, a steroid cream may be prescribed, but should be used with caution and for no more than 7 days (NHS QIS, 2010).

RTOG Score 2b and 3

There is insufficient evidence to suggest a definitive treatment for wet desquamation. The main goal is to choose a dressing that is comfortable for the patient and promotes healing. Depending on the level of exudate this could include hydrocolloids, hydrogels and silicone dressings, however, if radiotherapy treatment is still in progress and dressing removal is required for treatment it is best to avoid the use of adhesive dressings and/or tapes (NHS QIS, 2010). Grade 3 reactions may become infected, so should be observed daily. Infected reactions may be treated with antimicrobials, but dressings containing silver known to be absorbed into the tissues should not be used (NHS QIS, 210).

Care of the patient

The most important aspect of care of any patient undergoing radiotherapy must be communication. Written information can be used to reinforce verbal explanations. This provides the patient with a permanent record that can be shared with others. Information can help to allay anxiety for patients if they understand what is happening and know to expect some level of skin reaction. Although the UK radiotherapy centres in the UK provide written information for their patients, not all of the leaflets provide evidence-based information (Faithfull *et al.*, 2002). Hopefully, as hospitals seek to improve the information given to patients, this situation will change.

References

All Wales Tissue Viability Nurse Forum (2011) *Best Practice Statement: Assessment and Management of Skin Tears*. London: MA Healthcare Ltd, pp. 1–10.

Allami MK, Jamil W, Fourie B, Ashton V, Gregg PJ (2005) Superficial incisional infection in arthroplasty of the lower limb: interobserver reliability of the current diagnostic criteria. *Journal of Bone & Joint Surgery* (Br) **87**-B: 1267–1271.

Allen P (1996) Sternal wound dressings – a research study into risk factors. *British Journal of Theatre Nursing*, **6**: 38–39.

Alsbjörn B, Gilbert P, Hartmann B, Kaźmierski M, Monstrey S, Palao R, Roberto MA, van Trier A, Voinchet V (2007) Guidelines for the management of partial-thickness burns in a general hospital or community setting – recommendations of a European working party. *Burns*, **33**: 155–160.

Ashby E, Haddad FS, O'Donnell E, Wilson APR (2010) How will surgical site infection be measured to ensure "high quality care for all"? *Journal of Bone & Joint Surgery*, **92**: 1294–1299.

Atherton D, Sreetharan V, Mosahebi A, Prior S, Willis J, Bishop J, Dziewulski (2008) A randomised controlled trial of a double layer of Allevyn™ compared to Jelonet and proflavin as a tie-over dressing for small skin grafts. *Journal of Plastic, Reconstructive & Aesthetic Surgery*, **61**: 535–539.

Baier PK, Gluck NC, Baumgartner U, Adam U, Fischer A, Hopt UT (2010) Subcutaneous Redon drains do not reduce the incidence of surgical site infections after laparotomy. A randomised controlled trial in 200 patients. *International Journal of Colorectal Disease*, **25**: 639–643.

Bianchi J (2000) The cleansing of superficial traumatic wounds. *British Journal of Nursing*, **9** (suppl): S28–S36.

Bode LGM, Kluytmans JAJW, Wertheim HFL, Bogaers D, Vandenbroucke-Grauls CMJE, Rosendaal R, Troelstra A, Box ATA, Voss A, van der Tweel I, van Belkum A, Verbrugh HA, Vos MC (2010) Prevention surgical-site infections in nasal carriers of *Staphylococcus aureus*. *New England Journal of Medicine*, **362**: 9–17.

Campbell DA, Henderson WG, Englesbe MJ, Hall BL, O'Reilly M, Bratzler D, Dellinger EP, Neumayer L, Bass BL, Hutter MM, Schwartz J, Ko C, Itani K, Steinberg SM, Siperstein A, Sawyer RG, Turner DJ, Khuri SF (2008) Surgical site infection prevention: the importance of operative duration and blood transfusion – results of the first American College of Surgeons – national surgical quality improvement program best practices initiative. *Journal of the American College of Surgeons*, **207**: 810–820.

Chen E, Hornig S, Shepherd SM, Hollander JE (2000) Primary closure of mammalian bites. *Academic Emergency Medicine*, **7**: 157–161.

Chester DL, Jose RM, Aldlyami E, King H, Moieman NS (2006) Non-accidental burns in children – are we neglecting neglect? *Burns*, **32**: 222–228.

Chrintz H, Vibits H, Cordtz TO, Harreby JS, Waaddegaard P, Larsen SO (1989) Need for surgical wound dressing. *British Journal of Surgery*, **76**: 204–205.

Cohn SM, Gianotti G, Ong AW, Varela JE, Shatz DV, McKenney MG, Sleeman D, Ginzberg E, Augenstein JS, Byers PM, Sands LR, Hellinger MD, Namias N (2001) Prospective randomised trial of two wound management strategies for dirty abdominal wounds. *Annals of Surgery*, **233**: 409–413.

Collier M (1996) Trauma injury nursing in A&E. *Nursing Times*, **93**: 74–79.

Corion LUM, Smeulders MJC, van Zuijlen PPM, van der Horst CMAM (2009) Draining after breast reduction: a randomised controlled inter-patient study. *Journal of Plastic, Reconstructive & Aesthetic Surgery*, **62**: 865–868.

Coull A, Wylie K (1990) Regular monitoring: the way to ensure flap healing. *Professional Nurse*, **6**: 18–21.

Cox JD, Stetz J, Pajak TF (1995) Toxicity criteria of the Radiation Therapy Oncology Group (RTOG) and the European Organisation for Research and Treatment of Cancer (EORTC). *International Journal of Radiation Oncology, Biology & Physics*, **31**: 1341–1346.

Cruse PJE, Foord R (1980) The epidemiology of wound infection, a ten-year prospective study of 62,939 wounds. *Surgical Clinics of North America*, **60**: 27–40.

Cuttle L, Kimble RM (2010) First aid treatment of burn injuries. *Primary Intention*, **18**: 6–13.

Davey RB, Sparnon AL, Lodge M (2003) Technique of split skin graft fixation using hypafix: a 15-year review. *Australian & New Zealand Journal of Surgery*, **73**: 958–962.

Davis A, Chester D, Allison K, Davison P (2004) A survey of how a region's A&E units manage pretibial lacerations. *Journal of Wound Care*, **13**: 5–7.

Degraw M, Hicks RA, Lindberg D (2010) Incidence of fractures among children with burns with concern regarding abuse. Pediatrics, **125**: e295–e299.

Dendle C (2009) Management of mammalian bites. *Australian Family Physician*, **38**: 868–874.

Duttaroy DD, Jitendra J, Duttaroy B, Bansal U, Dhameja P, Patel G, Modi N (2009) Management strategy for dirty abdominal incisions: primary or delayed primary closure? A randomised trial. *Surgical Infections*, **10**: 129–136.

Dunkin CSJ, Elfleet D, Ling CA, La Hause Brown T (2003) A step by step guide to classifying and managing pretibial injuries. *Journal of Wound Care*, **12**: 109–111.

Edelman LS (2007) Social and economic factors associated with risk of burn injury. *Burns*, **33**: 958–965.

Edwards H, Gaskill D, Nash R (1998) Treating skin tears in nursing home residents: a pilot study comparing four types of dressings. International Journal of Nursing Practice, **4**: 25–32.

Enoch S, Roshan A, Shah M (2009) Emergency and early management of burns and scalds. *BMJ*, **338**: b1037.

Evans RC, Jones NL (1996) The management of abrasions and bruises. *Journal of Wound Care*, **5**: 465–468.

Eyal AS, Kemp M, Luvhengo T (2006) A 10-year audit of burns at Kalafong Hospital. *Burns*, **33**: 393–395.

Faithfull S, Hilton M, Booth K (2002) Survey of information leaflets on advice for acute radiation skin reactions in UK radiotherapy centres: a rationale for a systematic review of the literature. *European Journal of Oncology Nursing*, **6**: 176–178.

Farion K, Russell K, Osmond MH, Hartling L, Klassen T, Durec T, Vandermeer B (2009) Tissue adhesives for traumatic lacerations in children and adults. *Cochrane Database of Systematic Reviews*, **4**: CD003326.

Fowler A, Dempsey A (1998) Split-thickness skin graft donor sites. *Journal of Wound Care*, **7**: 399–402.

Fowler A (2003) The management of non-complex wounds within the community. *Nursing Times*, **99** (suppl): 5–7.

Francis A (1998) Nursing management of skin graft sites. *Nursing Standard*, **12**: 41–44.

Freedman BM, Oplinger EH, Freedman IS (2005) Topical becaplermin improves outcomes in work related fingertip injuries. *Journal of Trauma*, **59**: 965–968.

Gaine WJ, Andrew SM, Chadwick P, Cooke E, Bradley Williamson J (2001) Late operative site pain with Isola posterior instrumentation requiring implant removal. *Spine*, **26**: 583–587.

Gallico GG, O'Connor NE, Compton CC, Kehinde O, Green H (1984) Permanent cover of large burn wounds with autologous cultured human epithelium. *New England Journal of Medicine*, **311**: 448–451.

Gates S, Anderson ER (2010) Wound drainage for caesarean section. *Cochrane Database of Systematic Reviews*, **1**: CD004549.

Geary PM, Tiernan E (2009) Management of split skin graft donor sites – results of a national survey. *Journal of Plastic, Reconstructive & Aesthetic Surgery*, **62**: 1677–1683.

Gordon M, Goodwin CW (1997) Initial assessment, management and stabilisation. *Nursing Clinics of North America*, **32**: 237–249.

Grobler M, Kgosana R, Nsibande M, Phahlamohlaka M, Sefatsa P (2010) Skin care during breast radiotherapy. *South African Radiographer*, **48**: 15–17.

Gurusamy KS, Samraj K, Mullerat P, Davidson BR (2009) Routine abdominal drainage for uncomplicated open cholecystectomy. *Cochrane Database of Systematic Reviews*, **4**: CD006004.

Gurusamy KS, Samraj K (2009) Routine abdominal drainage for uncomplicated laproscopic cholecystectomy. *Cochrane Database of Systematic Reviews*, **2**: CD006003.

Harding KG (1990) Wound care: putting theory into clinical practice. In: Krasner D ed. *Chronic Wound Care*. Malvern, PA: Health Management Publications Inc.

Harrington G, Russo P, Spelman D, Borrell S, Watson K, Barr W, Martin R, Edmonds D, Cocks J, Greenbough J, Lowe J, Randle L, Castell J, Browne E, Bellis K, Aberline M (2004) Surgical-site infection rates and risk factor analysis in coronary artery bypass graft surgery. *Infection Control & Hospital Epidemiology*, **25**: 472–476.

Heal C, Buettner P, Raasch B, Browning S, Graham D, Bidgood R, Campbell M, Cruikshank R (2006) Can sutures get wet? Prospective randomised controlled trial of wound management in general practice. *British Medical Journal*, **332**: 1053–1056.

Health Protection Agency (2009) *Healthcare-Associated Infections in England: 2008–2009 Report*. HPA, London.

Heggie S, Bryant GP, Tripcony L, Keller J, Rose P, Glendenning M, Heath J (2002) A phase III study on the efficacy of aloe vera gel on irradiated breast tissue. *Cancer Nursing*, **25**: 442–451.

Hermans MHE (2007) Results of an internet survey on the treatment of partial thickness burns, full thickness burns and donor sites. *Journal of Burn Care Research*, **28**: 835–847.

Hettiaratchy S, Dziewulski P (2004a) ABC of Burns: Pathophysiology and types of burns. *British Medical Journal*, **328**: 1427–1430.

Hettiaratchy S, Dziewulski P(2004b) ABC of Burns: Introduction. *British Medical Journal*, **328**: 1366–1368.

Hettiaratchy S, Papini R (2004) ABC of Burns: Initial management of a major burn: I – overview. *British Medical Journal*, **328**: 1555–1557.

Higgins MAG, Evans RC, Evans RJ (1997) Managing animal bite wounds. *Journal of Wound Care*, **6**: 377–380.

Holm C, Pederson JS, Gronbaek F, Gottrup F (1998) Effects of occlusive and conventional gauze dressings on incisional healing after abdominal operations. *European Journal of Surgery*, **164**: 179–183.

James-Ellison M, Barnes P, Maddocks A, Wareham K, Drew P, Dickson W, Lyons RA, Hutchings H (2009) Social health outcomes following thermal injuries: a retrospective matched cohort study. *Archives of Diseases of Childhood*, **94**: 663–667.

Jonkers D, Elenbaas T, Terporten P, Nieman F, Stobberingh E (2003) Prevalence of 90-days postoperative wound infections after cardiac surgery. *European Journal of Cardiothoracic Surgery*, **23**: 97–102.

Khan MN, Naqvi AH (2006) Antiseptics, iodine, povidone iodine and traumatic wound cleansing. *Journal of Tissue Viability*, **16**: 6–10.

Knaust A, Moussa M, Stilianakis NI, Eikmann T, Herr C (2009) Three questions to screen for post discharge surgical site infections. *American Journal of Infection Control*, **37**: 420–422.

Lawrence JC, Wilkins MD (1986) *The Epidemiology of Burns*. In: Burncare Symposium at Birmingham University, April 1986..

Leaper DJ, van Goor H, Reilly J, Pertosillo N, Geiss HK, Torres AJ, Berger A (2004) Surgical site infection – a European perspective of incidence and economic burden. *International Wound Journal*, **1**: 247–273.

Ljungberg E, Rosberg HE, Dahlin LB (2003) Hand injuries in young children. *Journal of Hand Surgery (British Volume)*, **28B**: 376–380.

Lund CC, Browder NC (1944) Estimations of areas of burns. *Surgery, Gynaecology and Obstetrics*, **79**: 352.

Lyall PW, Sinclair SW (2000) Australasian survey of split skin graft donor sites. *Australian & New Zealand Surgery*, **70**: 114–116.

Ma KK, Chan MF, Pang SMC (2006) The effectiveness of using a lipido-colloid dressing for patients with traumatic digital wounds. *Clinical Nursing Research*, **15**: 119–134.

McGough-Csarny J, Kopac CA (1998) Objectives 1: risk factor identification. Skin tears in institutionalised elderly: an epidemiological study. *Ostomy & Wound Management*, **44** (suppl): 14S–25S.

McQuestion M (2006) Evidence-based skin care management in radiation therapy. *Seminars in Oncology Nursing*, **22**: 163–173.

Medeiros I, Saconato H (2001) Antibiotic prophylaxis for mammalian bites. *The Cochrane Library*, **2**: CD001738.

Meuleneire F (2002) Using a soft silicone-coated net dressing to manage skin tears. *Journal of Wound Care*, **11**: 365–369.

Mileski WJ, Atiles L, Purdue G, Kagan R, Saffle JR, Herndon DN, Heimbach D, uterman A, Yurt R, Goodwin C, Hunt JL (2003) Serial measurements increase the accuracy of laser Doppler assessment of burn wounds. *Journal of Burn Care & Rehabilitation*, **24**: 187–191.

Moisidis E, Heath T, Boorer C, Ho K, Deva AK (2004) A prospective, blinded, randomised, controlled clinical trial of topical negative pressure use in skin grafting. *Plastic & Reconstructive Surgery*, **114**: 917–922.

Molina JE, Lew R S-L, Hyland KJ (2004) Postoperative sternal dehiscence in obese patients: incidence and prevention. *Annals of Thoracic Surgery*, **78**: 912–917.

Muneuchi G, Tamai M, Igawa K, Kurokawa M, Igawa HH (2005) The PNB classification for treatment of fingertip injuries: the boundary between conservative treatment and surgical treatment. *Annals of Plastic Surgery*, **54**: 604–609.

Murphy F (2006) Assessment and management of patients with surgical cavity wounds. *Nursing Standard*, **20**: 57–66.

National Burn Care Review Committee (NBCRC) (2001) *Standards and Strategy for Burn Care: A Review of Burn Care in the British Isles*. London: NBCRC.

National Institute for Health and Clinical Excellence (2008) *Surgical Site Infection: Prevention and Treatment of Surgical Site Infection*. London: NICE.

National Institute for Health and Clinical Excellence (2009) *Clinical Guideline 89: When to suspect child maltreatment*. London: NICE.

New South Wales Health (2008) *Burn Transfer Guidelines – NSW Severe Burn Injury Service*, 2nd edn. North Sydney: NSW Health.

NHS Quality Improvement Scotland (2010) *Best Practice Statement: Skincare of Patients Receiving Radiotherapy*. Edinburgh: NHS QIS.

NHS Choices (2011) Burns and Scalds. London: NHS Choices (http://www.nhs.uk/conditions/burns-and-scalds/pages/introduction.aspx).

Nienhuijs SW, Manupassa R, Strobbe LJA, Rosman C (2003) Can topical negative pressure be used to control complex enterocutaneous fistulae? *Journal of Wound Care*, **12**: 343–345.

Parker MJ, Livingstone V, Clifton R, McKee A (2008) Closed suction surgical wound drainage after orthopaedic surgery. *Cochrane Database of Systematic Reviews*, **3**: CD001825.

Payne RL, Martin MC (1993) Defining and classifying skin tears: need for a common language. A criticque and revision of the Payne-Martin classification system for skin tears. *Ostomy & Wound Management*, **39**: 16–26.

Prelack K, Dylewski M, Sheridan RL (2007) Practical guidelines for nutritional management of burn injury and recovery. *Burns*, **33**: 14–24.

Roh MR, Shin J-U, Chung KY (2008) Slicone net bolster dressing for skin grafts. *Dermatologic Surgery*, **14**: 1233–1235.

Salvo N, Barnes E, van Draanen J, Stacey E, Mitera G, Breen D, Giotis A, Czarnota G, Pang J, De Angelis C (2010) Prophylaxis and management of acute radiation-induced skin reactions: a systematic review of the literature. *Current Oncology*, **17**: 94–112.

Samraj K, Gurusamy KS (2008) Wound drains following thyroid surgery. *Cochrane Database of Systematic Reviews*, **4**: CD006099.

Shetty AA, Kumar VS, Morgan-Hough C, Georgeu GA, James KD, Nicholl JE (2004) Comparing wound complication rates following closure of hip wounds with metallic skin stapes or subcuticular vivryl suture: a prospective randomised trial. *Journal of Orthopaedic Surgery*, **12**: 191–193.

Singer AJ, Hollander JE, Quinn JV (1997) Evaluation and management of traumatic lacerations. *New England Journal of Medicine*, **337**: 1142–1148.

Tanner J, Woodings D, Moncaster K (2008) Preoperative hair removal to reduce surgical site infection. *Cochrane Database of Systematic Reviews*, **3**: CD004122.

Thomas DR, Goode PS, LaMaster K, Tennyson T, Parnell LKS (1999) A comparison of an opaque foam dressing versus a transparent film dressing in the management of skin tears in institutionalised subjects. *Ostomy & Wound Management*, **45**: 22–28.

Thombs BD (2008) Patient and injury characteristics, mortality risk and length of stay related to child abuse by burning. *Annals of Surgery*, **247**: 519–523.

Vermeulen H, Ubbink D, Goossens A, de Vos R, Legemate D, Westerbos SJ (2010) Dressings and topical agents for surgical wounds healing by secondary intention. *Cochrane Database of Systematic Reviews*, **1**: CD003554.

Vilar-Compte D, Rosales S, Hernandez-Mello N, Maafs E (2009) Surveillance, control and prevention of surgical site infections in breast cancer surgery: a 5-year experience. *American Journal of Infection Control*, **37**: 674–679.

Voineskos SH, Ayeni OA, McNight L, Thoma A (2009) Systematic review of skin graft donor sites. *Plastic & Reconstructive Surgery*, **124**: 298–306.

Wallace AB (1951) The exposure treatment of burns. *Lancet*, **i**: 501–504.

Webster J, Osborne S (2011) Preoperative bathing or showering with skin antiseptics to prevent surgical site infection. *Cochrane Database of Systematic Reviews*, **2**: CD004985.

Weiss Y (1983) Simplified management of operative wounds by early exposure. *International Surgery*, **68**: 237–240.

Wells M, Macmillan M, Raab G, MacBride S, Bell N, MacKinnon K, MacDougall H, Samual L, Munro A (2004) Does aqueous or sucralfate cream affect the severity of erythematous radiation skin reactions? A randomised controlled trial. *Radiotherapy & Oncology*, **73**: 153–162.

Westaby S (1985) Wound closure and drainage. In Westaby S ed. *Wound Care*. London: William Heineman Medical Books Ltd.

Whaley S (2004) Tap water or normal saline for cleansing traumatic wounds? *British Journal of Community Nursing*, **9**: 471–478.

Wiechula R (2003) The use of moist wound healing dressings in the management of split-thickness skin graft donor sites: a systematic review. *International Journal of Nursing Practice*, **9** (suppl): S9–S17.

Wikblad K, Anderson B (1995) A comparison of three wound dressings in patients undergoing heart surgery. *Nursing Research*, **44**: 312–316.

Wilkinson B (1997) Hard graft. *Nursing Times*, **93**: 63–68.

Wilson AP, Ward VP, Coello R, Charlett A, Pearson A (2002) A user evaluation of the Nosocomial Infection National Surveillance Scheme surgical site infection module. *Journal of Hospital Infection*, **52**: 114–121.

Wilson APR, Weavill C, Burridge J, Kelsey MC (1990) The use of the wound scoring method 'ASEPSIS' in postoperative wound surveillance. *Journal of Hospital Infection*, **16**: 297–300.

Wynne R, Botti M, Stedman H, Holsworth L (2004) Effect of three wound dressings on infection, healing comfort and cost in patients with sternotomy wounds: a randomised trial. *Chest*, **125**: 43–50.

Yeo CJ, Sebastion SJ, Chong AKS (2010) Fingertip injuries. *Singapore Medicine*, **51**: 78–87.

7 The Organisation of Wound Management

Introduction

The organisation of the delivery of wound care has undergone great change in the last few years. This chapter will be exploring some of the aspects of wound care delivery that have had a great impact on nurses and nursing, both in the hospital and in the community. Overall, these changes have ensured that patients have received more effective care.

Managing wounds in the community

In earlier chapters of this book the prevalence of various types of wounds has been described, but it is useful to consider the overall burden of wounds across patient populations in the community. A number of prevalence surveys have been undertaken, but it is difficult to make comparisons because of the different methodologies used, but it is interesting to look at the variations across different populations.

In India, Gupta *et al.* (2004) surveyed an urban and an adjacent rural community and found a wound prevalence of 15.03:1000. There were just over twice as many acute wounds as chronic wounds and the commonest site for both was on the lower extremity. The commonest aetiology for the chronic wounds on the leg or foot was that of an untreated, non-healing traumatic injury. A prevalence survey undertaken in Ireland found a crude prevalence of 15.6% but the most frequent wounds were pressure ulcers (McDermott-Scales *et al.*, 2009).

Two other surveys, both undertaken in the north of England, have looked at both acute and community sectors. Srinivasaiah *et al.* (2007) found an overall prevalence of 12%, but also found that community nurses were involved in caring for 70.1% of the patients with wounds. They found surgical wounds to be the most common wound type, although it is not clear if this is because of the impact of including hospital patients in the survey. Vowden and Vowden (2009a) found a prevalence of 3.55 people with wounds per 1000 population. Of the 1735 people with wounds,

The Care of Wounds: A Guide for Nurses, Fourth Edition. Carol Dealey.
© 2012 Carol Dealey. Published 2012 by John Wiley & Sons, Ltd.

68% were being cared for in a variety of care settings such as their own home or a residential or nursing home. Again, the commonest wound type were acute wounds across all the populations, making it difficult to determine the precise situation in the community. However, of the 826 people with acute wounds, 382 (46.2%) were being cared for in their own homes or in general practitioner surgeries (Vowden & Vowden 2009b).

The dominant finding from these surveys is that nurses working in the community are required to provide care for patients with a wide variety of wounds. It therefore follows that they need skills in wound management and access to expert advice.

Nurse specialists in wound care

Specialist nurses in wound care have a variety of titles, but the most common in the UK is that of clinical nurse specialist in tissue viability (TVN). They straddle both hospital and community as TVN may be found in both community and hospital trusts. It is a relatively new nursing speciality developed in the late 1980s and the numbers have grown rapidly. The precise number is difficult to determine as there is no formal register, however Finnie (2004) suggested that there were around 500 in post as well as a few nurse consultants.

Education is an essential prerequisite for the recognition of any speciality. Fletcher (1998) found that there are a variety of courses available within the UK. They comprise short courses at diploma level as well as degree- and masters-level programmes. Fairbairn (2001) discussed the potential for a clinical doctorate for TVNs as an alternative to undertaking a PhD following the more traditional route. He suggested that this option is more flexible allowing the student to utilise aspects of existing work. A more recent development has been that of a competency framework devised for TVNs in Scotland, but it is intended for wider use (Finnie & Wilson, 2003). It involves six domains: clinical problem-solving, professional practice, teamwork, reflective practice, empowerment and leadership.

Austin (2002) undertook a survey of TVNs in one region of the UK and found several clearly defined aspects of the role.

- *Clinical role*: all the TVNs had direct clinical contact with patients, receiving referrals predominantly from nurses.
- *Educator role*: this is an important aspect of the role. The survey found that TVNs mostly taught nurses, but they also taught other disciplines such as doctors, allied health professionals and social workers.
- *Leadership role*: all respondents had a remit that extended across their organisation involving advice on purchasing or commissioning resources (94%) standards or guideline development (93%); and audit of care provision (83%).

- *Research role*: 57% had participated in research, predominantly product evaluations. This aspect of the role generally requires further development (Gray, 2004).
- *Management role*: respondents indicated that it involved managing a team (39%) and/or holding the service budget (42%) or influencing the budget expenditure.

Austin's survey provides a picture of TVN activity that is fairly representative. She also noted that the role is poorly understood by others. Flanagan (1996) described some of the difficulties that the TVN may face. They include unrealistic objectives or targets, role ambiguity, responsibilities across large geographical areas or multiple sites, constant pressure to reduce the cost of the tissue viability service and often having to work with insufficient resources with limited professional support. Although written some time ago, little seems to have changed for present-day TVN.

Despite the constraints the role of the TVN still presents the post holder with considerable opportunities to enhance nursing practice and the personal satisfaction in seeing wounds healing and patients' quality of life improve.

Multiprofessional wound care

Wound care is not just a nursing activity, but requires a multiprofessional approach. The relevant disciplines include: nursing, medicine, dietetics, podiatry, physiotherapy and occupational therapy. To date, there has been limited interest in wound care from doctors and little in their training that might stimulate such an interest (Ennis *et al.*, 2004). Podiatrists have focused mainly on diabetic foot problems and other disciplines have had varied levels of interest in wounds. Yet using a multiprofessional approach is not only effective in terms of improved patient outcomes, it also has the potential to provide cost savings. Vu *et al.* (2007) undertook a pseudo-randomised pragmatic cluster trial in nursing homes in Melbourne, Australia comparing standardised treatment from a wound care team with usual care. They found significantly increased healing rates and lower costs for those treated by the wound care team.

The main problem for many members of a wound care team is that wound care is only a small part of their work, rather than their main focus. For wound care to become a recognised specialty there needs to be adequate education, especially for medical doctors. Education to Master's degree level is available in a number of countries, most courses being open to all disciplines and in the USA it is possible to undertake a course and examination to become a certified wound specialist.

Ennis *et al.* (2004) proposed a medical fellowship in wound care for doctors wishing to become a full-time consultant in wound care. Such a training programme would take 18 months and include a mixture of theoretical and clinical work. For those with specialist surgical training there would be specific medical skill-sets to learn and vice versa for those with medical training. This is a very interesting proposal, but would only be practical in a facility with a wound healing centre.

Wound healing centres

Wound healing centres started in the USA and there are now many established across the country, many of them commercially run. They are less common elsewhere, but gradually a few centres are starting in Europe, in particular in the UK and Denmark. The most important aspect of effective care provision within wound clinics is the multidisciplinary approach and access to other specialties as required (Gottrup, 2004b).

Although the centres all function differently, they have a number of common features.

- The staff working in wound healing centres includes a variety of healthcare professionals. The range of professionals varies from centre to centre.
- Most are based within teaching hospitals and provide education pro- grammes of varying types.
- Some treat both inpatients and outpatients, referred from both the primary and secondary healthcare sectors, although the number of inpatient beds may be limited.
- The centres treat a variety of complex wounds, not jut one wound type.
- All the wound healing centres are involved in research programmes.

Beyond this common ground the centres all function differently, due to the circumstances in which they were developed. The centres in Denmark have been fully integrated into the national health service allowing for country-wide referrals. Gottrup (2004a) suggests that for Denmark with its 5.2 million inhabitants, only one or two clinics are necessary. Obviously larger or more densely populated countries would require more centres to provide the same levels of care provision.

Wound healing centres have a great deal to offer in terms of specialised care for problem wounds; educational opportunities to increase the num- bers of clinical staff with specialist knowledge and an important research function to assist in developing the evidence base for this important subject.

Conclusions

Wound care is increasingly being recognised as an important aspect of nursing care and it is becoming ever more sophisticated. Despite this, there are still areas of poor practice and patients who receive less than optimum care. It is hoped that these variations in practice will decrease as more evidence and more guidelines become available to guide the practitioner.

References

Austin L (2002) A survey of tissue viability nurses' role and background in one region. *Journal of Wound Care*, **11**: 347–350.

Ennis WJ, Valdes W, Meneses P (2004) Wound care specialisation: a proposal for a comprehensive fellowship program. *Wound Repair & Regeneration*, **12**: 120–128.

Fairbairn G (2001) The role of a clinical doctorate in the advancement of practice. *British Journal of Nursing*, **10** (suppl): S4–S5.

Finnie A (2004) We must act to move tissue viability forward. *British Journal of Nursing*, **13** (suppl): S3.

Finnie A, Wilson A (2003) Development of a tissue viability nursing competency framework. *British Journal of Nursing*, **12** (suppl): S38–S44.

Flanagan, M. (1996) The role of the clinical nurse specialist in tissue viability. *British Journal of Nursing*, **5**: 676–681.

Fletcher J (1998) A survey of courses available that are relevant to the field of tissue viability. In: Leaper D, Dealey C, Franks PJ, Hofman D, Moffatt C eds. *Proceedings of the 7th European Conference on Advances in Wound Management*. London: EMAP Healthcare Ltd.

Gottrup F (2004a) A specialised wound-healing centre concept: importance of a multidisciplinary department structure and surgical treatment facilities in the treatment of chronic wounds. *American Journal of Surgery*, **187** (suppl): 38S–43S.

Gottrup F (2004b) Optimising wound treatment through health care structuring and professional education. *Wound Repair & Regeneration*, **12**: 129–133.

Gray D (2004) Specialists must accept challenge of improving clinical outcomes. *British Journal of Nursing*, **13** (suppl): S4.

Gupta N, Gupta SK, Shukla VK, Singh SP (2004) An Indian community-based epidemiological study of wounds. *Journal of Wound Care*, **13**: 323–325.

McDermott-Scales L, Cowman S, Gethin G (2009) Prevalence of wounds in a community setting in Ireland. *Journal of Wound Care*, **18**: 405–417.

Srinivasaiah N, Dugdall H, Barrett S, Drew PJ (2007) A point prevalence survey of wounds in north-east England. *Journal of Wound Care*, **16**: 413–416.

Vowden KR, Vowden P (2009a) A survey of wound care provision within one English health care district. *Journal of Tissue Viability*, **18**: 2–6.

Vowden KR, Vowden P (2009b) The prevalence, management and outcome for acute wounds identified in a wound care survey within one English health care district. *Journal of Tissue Viability*, **18**: 7–12.

Vu T, Harris A, Duncan G, Sussman G (2007) Cost-effectiveness of multidisciplinary wound care in nursing homes: a pseudo-randomised pragmatic cluster trial. *Family Practice*, **24**: 372–379.

Index

Page numbers in *italics* denote figures, those in **bold** denote tables.

ABCDEF assessment in burns care   212
abrasions   201
absorbent dressings   110–11
acute wounds   62, 185–226
   burns   205–16
   radiation reactions   216–19
   surgical   185–99
   traumatic   199–205
adherent dressings   172, 203
   see also low-adherent dressings
adhesive island dressings   186
adrenocorticotrophic hormone (ACTH)   28
ageing effects *see* elderly people
alginate dressings   113, 188
   abrasions   201
   chronic wounds   155
   donor sites   190
   leg ulcers   155
   moist wound healing   79, 80, 83
   necrotic/sloughing wounds   197
   oozing wounds   147
   sloughing wounds   155
   surgical wounds   187, 188
alginate rope   187
allergy to dressings   77, *78*
alternative therapies   41
animal bites   203–4
ankle brachial pressure index   154
antibiotics   21, 82, 102, 107, 115, 169, **170**, 173, **194**, 195, 200, 202, 203
antimicrobial dressings   113–14
antiseptics   102–7
   rarely used   105–7
   widely used   103–5
anxiety   39–41
Apligraf   119–20
appearance of wounds   69–75

diabetic ulcers   167–9, **168**
   pressure ulcers   143–6
   venous leg ulcers   152–4, *153*, **153**
aromatherapy   41
arterial leg ulcers   159–65
   aetiology   159–60
   management   160–5
ASEPSIS wound scoring system   193, *194*
aseptic procedures   101
assessment of wounds
   burns   212–13
   diabetic ulcers   167–9, **168**
   minor trauma   199–201
   pressure ulcers   143–6
   surgical wounds   185–6
   venous leg ulcers   152–4, *153*, **153**
atherosclerosis   159
audit   18, 74, 192, 228
autolytic debridement   80

bag systems   83
bandages   36, 42, 67, 83, 93, 96, 98, 99, 100, 151, 154, 156
barrier-film dressings   115
basal cell carcinoma   163–4
bed sores *see* pressure ulcers
beds, pressure-relieving   140–1
betaine   104
biofilm infections   21, 71–2
biosurgery *see* larval therapy
bite wounds   203–4
bleeding *see* haemorrhage
blood supply   134–5
body image   41–2
body temperature   **136**, 208
bolster dressings   189
Braden score   136, **136**

The Care of Wounds: A Guide for Nurses, Fourth Edition. Carol Dealey.
© 2012 Carol Dealey. Published 2012 by John Wiley & Sons, Ltd.

British Association for Parenteral and Enteral
    Nutrition (BAPEN) 19
British Pharmaceutical Codices 100
Buerger's disease 160
burn wounds 17, 75, 205–16
    aetiology 206–7
    aftercare 216
    complex 212
    deep dermal/full-thickness 216
    depth **214**
    first aid 208–9
    incidence 207–8
    non-complex 212–13
    nutrition 213
    oedema 210–11, *211*
    patient assessment 213
    Rule of Nines *210*
    severity 209–10, *210*
    superficial burns 313
    superficial dermal 214–16, *215*
    wound assessment 213

cadexemer iodine 103
cancer patients 22
    anxiety 42
    fungating wounds 170–1
    pain relief 33
    radiotherapy 38–9
    spiritual care 45–6
capillary action dressings 113
capillary pressure 130
carbohydrates **20**
carbolic acid 99
care environment 63
cavity wounds 8, 75
    antiseptics 106, 107
    dressings 63, 112, 113
    granulating 73
    pressure ulcers 146, 148
cetrimide 105
chairs, pressure sores 139–40
chemotherapeutic drugs 23
child abuse 208
chlorhexidine 105
chronic wounds 11–12, 61,
    127–83
    diabetic ulcers 165–70
    fungating 170–4

leg ulcers 149–65
pressure ulcers 127–49
classification of wounds 61–2
cleansing wounds 66, 69, 85, 94,
    96, 100
    antiseptics 104–5
    burns 214
    lotions 102
    pain caused by 75
    pressure ulcers 142
    saline 107–8
    tap water 108
    venous leg ulcers 155
clinical guidelines
    diabetic ulcers **170**
    hand hygiene 24
    leg ulcers 152
    MRSA 107
    nursing interventions 19–20, 23
    nutrition 15, 18, 19
    palliative care 45
    pressure ulcers 148–9
    sleep promotion 35
    traumatic wounds 200
clinical nurse specialists 228
closed wounds 2
clotting cascade 4
collagenase 20
commitment 48
communication 31, **46**, 127, 219
community management 227–8
complement system 4
compression 83
    leg ulcers 156
    pneumatic 157
compression stockings 156–7
contact dermatitis *78*
contact inhibition 8
contractures 10–11
copper **20**
costs of healing
    chronic wounds 127
    dressings 87
    leg ulcers 150–1
    pressure ulcers 128, 147–8
cotton wool 99
crushing finger-tip injuries 202–3
cushions 141

Dakin's solution   99, 106
debridement   98
  autolytic   80
  enzymatic   80, 82
  larval therapy   80
  mechanical   82
  surgical   82
decubitus ulcers *see* pressure ulcers
definitions   1–2
dehiscence   196–7, *197*
delayed primary closure   99, 187
depth of wounds   62, 64, 66
  abrasions   201
  burns   213, **214**
  pressure ulcers   144
Dermagraft   119–20
dermatitis
  contact   *78*
  incontinence-associated   142, 144,
      145, 146
dermis   2
diabetes mellitus   26–7
diabetic ulcers   165–70
  aetiology   166
  assessment   167–9, **168**, *169*
  clinical guidelines   **170**
  management   167–70
  prevention   166–7
digital image analysis   65
drainage of legs   155–6
drains   191–2
dressing changes   75
dressings   93–126
  absorbent   110–11
  adherent   172, 203
  advanced   111–13
  allergy to   77, *78*
  antimicrobial   113–14
  cavity wounds   63, 112, 113
  clinical effectiveness   108–10
  conformability   109
  cost   87
  cost of   87
  ease of application   87, 109
  effectiveness   87
  epithelialising wounds   73, *73*
  granulating wounds   72–3, *73*
  handling qualities   109

  history   93–100
  infected wounds   70–2, *70*
  leg ulcers   155
  necrotic wounds   69, *69*
  patient comfort   86–7, 109
  skin graft donor sites   190–1
  skin protection   115
  specialised   114
  surgical wounds   187–8
  traditional   100–1
  wound contact   110–11
  see also individual types

eating *see* nutrition
elastase   20
elderly people
  burns   17, 207
  leg ulcers   150
  nutrition   18
  pressure ulcers   131, 133, 138
  skin tears   204
  special needs of   19
emollients   142, 191
empathy   48
Emplastrums   100
enzymatic debridement   80, 82
epidermal growth factor   **5**, 8
epidermis   3
epithelialisation   8, 73, *73*
erosion   62
eschar   1
ESCHAR study   159
Eupad   100
European Society for Clinical Nutrition and
      Metabolism (ESPEN)   19
European Tissue Repair Society   85
exudate   67–8, **68**, 173

fats   **20**
fear   43
fibrinolysin   20
fibroblast growth factor   **5**
fibroblasts   7
  premature ageing   12
fibronectin   5–6, 7
finger-tip injuries   202–3
first intention healing   2, 8, 186
fistulae   198–9

flap (pedicle) grafts   188
foam dressings   112–13
    burn injuries   216
    burns   216
    leg ulcers   155
    pressure ulcers   147
foot ulcers *see* diabetic ulcers
full-thickness burns   216
full-thickness wounds   2, 62
Functional Assessment of Chronic Illness
        Therapy-Spiritual Well-Being
        (FACIT-sp)   33
fungating wounds   170–4
    aetiology and incidence   170–1
    management   171–4
    quality of life   171

gauze dressings   189
glucocorticoids   28, 37, 38
granulation   72–3, *73*
grief   43
growth factors   **5**
growth hormone   34

haemorrhage
    fungating wounds   172
    surgical wounds   192
Hageman factor   4
hair, shaving   23
hand hygiene   24–5
    clinical guidelines   24
healing   3–9
    epithelialisation   8
    first intention   2, 8, 186
    impaired   9–12
    inflammation   4–6, **4**, **5**
    maturation   9
    moist   79
    physiology of   1–14
    reconstruction   6–8
    second intention   2, 187–92
highly absorbent dressings   83
honey   104, 114
hospitals
    mattresses   140–1
    pressure-relieving equipment
        139–41
    sleep disturbance   34–6, 213

HSE (human skin equivalents)   120
humility, nursing staff   48
hydrocolloids   20, 112
    autolytic debridement   80
    leg ulcers   155
    minor trauma   201, 205
    odour from   68
    pressure ulcers   147
    skin donor sites   190
    surgical wounds   186
hydrogels   20, 111
    autolytic debridement   80
    burn injuries   216
    leg ulcers   115, 155
    minor trauma   202
    sinuses   198
hydrogen peroxide   105–6
hyperbaric oxygen   117–18
Hyperfix   189
hypertrophic scars   9–10
hypothermia   36–7

impaired wound healing   9–12
    chronic wounds   11–12
    contractures   10–11
    hypertrophic scars   9–10
    keloids   10
incontinence-associated dermatitis   142, 144,
        145, 146
infection   21–5, 70–2, *70*
    control of   82–3
    nursing interventions   23–5
    risk factors
        age   22
        length of pre-operative stay   23
        nutritional status   22
        obesity   22
        shaving   23
        smoking   23
        type of surgery   23
        underlying illness   22
    skin grafts   190
    surgical wounds   192–6, **193**, *194*
inflammation   4–6, **5**, 82–3
insulin-like growth factors   **5**
iodine   99, 103, 114
iron   **20**
irritant dermatitis   *78*

keloids   10
kinin system   4
knitted viscose dressings   110

lacerations   201–2
larval therapy   80, 115
leg ulcers   149–65
  aetiology   151
  arterial   159–65
  clinical guidelines   152
  cost of   150–1
  diabetic *see* diabetic ulcers
  dressings   155
  epidemiology   149–50
  evaluation   158
  malignant   163–4
  mixed aetiology   162–3
  prevention of recurrence   158–9
  rheumatoid arthritis   164–5
  skin care   155
  skin grafts   155
  venous   151–60, 161
lifting patients   135
lint   99
lipodermatosclerosis   152
listening to patients   48
lotions   102–8
  antibiotics   107
  antiseptics   102–7
  saline   107
  tap water   108
low-adherent dressings   110, 113, 155, 173,
     202, 204
Lund & Browder chart, burn injuries   *211*
lymphocytes   6
lymphoedema   164

macrophages   6–7
maggots *see* larval therapy
malignant fungating wounds   170–1
malignant leg ulcers   163–4
malnutrition   16
mast cells   6
matrix metalloproteinases   7, 21, 72
mattresses   140–1
maturation   9
MEASURE framework   **62**, 63–77
measurement of wounds   63–7

linear   64
surface area   64–6
volume   66–7
mechanical debridement   82
melanocytes   3
Mesalt   173
Mini-Nutritional Assessment
     Tool   18
mobility, reduced   131–2
moist wound healing   79
moisture balance   83–4
multiprofessional care   229–30
mupirocin   107
music therapy   41
myofibroblasts   7–8

necrosis   69, *69*
neurological deficit   133–4
neuropathic ulcers *see* diabetic ulcers
neutrophils   5–6
nurse specialists   228–9
nutrition   15–21, **20**
  burn patients   213
  nursing interventions   19–20
  outcomes monitoring   20–1
nutritional assessment   137
nutritional status   16–19
  and infection   22
  and infection risk   22
  and pressure ulcers   132–3

obesity   22
odour problems   68, **68**, 173
odour-absorbent dressings   113
oedema in burn wounds
     210–11, *211*
open wounds   2
overlays   140–1
oxygen, hyperbaric   117–18

pain   28–33, 75
  assessment   *16*, 31, *32, 33*
  attitudes to   29–30
  cause   32
  pressure ulcers   147
pain chart   *32*
pain management   84–5
  ABCD guide   31–3, *32, 33*

pain management (*Continued*)
  inadequate knowledge of health
      professionals   30
  time management   30
palliative care, pressure ulcers   148–9
paraffin gauze *see* tulle dressings
partial-thickness wounds   2, 62
patient management   15–60
  physical care   15–39
  psychological care   39–44
  spiritual care   45–8
pedicle (flap) grafts   188
pentoxifylline   158
peripheral neuropathy   166, 168
physical care   15–39
  diabetes mellitus   26–7
  hypothermia   36–7
  infection   21–5
  nutrition   15–21
  pain   28–33
  radiotherapy   38–9
  sleep disturbance   34–6
  smoking   25–6
  steroids   37–8
  stress   27–8
physiology of wound healing   1–14
pinch grafts   188
plastic surgery   148
platelet-derived growth factor   **5**
pneumatic compression   157
polyhexamethylene biguanide   104–5
polyurethane-matrix dressings   112
position of wound   63
post-operative wounds   62
potassium permanganate   106
povidone iodine   103
powerlessness   43–4
pressure ulcers   127–49
  aetiology   130–5
  assessment   143–6
  classification   143–6
  definition   128
  education and training   142
  elderly people   131, 133, 138
  location of   146–7
  management   143–9
  nutrition   137, 142
  pain assessment   147

palliative care   148–9
patient positioning   138–9
plastic surgery   148
prevalence and incidence   129
prevention   135, 137–43
risk assessment   136–7
seating   139–40
skin care   137, 141–2
support surfaces   140–1
wound bed   147
pressure-relieving devices   141
proflavine   106
protease-modulating dressings   114
protein   **20**
Pseudomonas aeruginosa   190
psychological care   39–44, 213
  anxiety   39–41
  body image   41–2
  fear   43
  grief   43
  powerlessness   43–4

radiation reactions   216–19
  aetiology   216–17
  classification   217
  management   218–19
  patient care   219
  prevention   217–18
radiotherapy   38–9
re-evaluation   76–7
reconstruction   6–8
repositioning of patients   138–9
rheumatoid leg ulcers   164–5
Rule of Nines, burn injuries   *210*

saline   107
scabbing   1
scars, hypertrophic   9–10
seating   139–40
second intention healing   2, 187–92
sensory deficit   133–4
shaving as infection risk   23
silicone keloid dressings   114
silicone net dressings   216
silver nitrate   104
silver sulphadiazine   103
silver-coated dressings   103–4, 114
sinus formation   197–8

skin   2–3, *3*
   age-related changes   133
   dermis   2
   epidermis   3
   moisture   134
skin assessment   137
   pressure ulcers   137
   venous leg ulcers   154
skin cancer   163
skin care   141–2
   leg ulcers   155
   pressure ulcers   137, 141–2
skin grafts   188–90
   donor sites   190–1
   failure of   190
   leg ulcers   155
skin tears   204–5, **205**
sleep disturbance   34–6, 213
   interventions   35–6
slough   72, *72*
smoking   25–6
   and infection risk   23
sodium hypochlorite   106–7
soft-polymer dressings   112
Sorbsan   87
spiritual care   45–8, **46**
squamous cell carcinoma   163–4
Staphylococcus aureus   195–6
State Trait Anxiety Inventory
      (STAI-State)   40
sterilisers   101
steroids   37–8
stratum basale   3
stratum corneum   3
stratum granulosum   3
stratum lucidum   3
stratum spinosum   3
stress   27–8
suffering   75
superficial wounds   62
support surfaces   140–1
surface area   64–6
surgical debridement   82
surgical site infection   192–6,
      193, *194*
surgical toilet   201
surgical wounds   185–99
   dehiscence   196–7, *197*

first intention healing   186
   delayed   187
fistula formation   198–9
haemorrhage   192
patient assessment   185
second intention healing   187–92
sinus formation   197–8
wound assessment   185–6

T lymphocytes   6
TELER exudate indicator   **68**
TIME framework   80, 82
TIMPs   10–11, 21
tissue adhesives   201
tissue culture   118–19, 188–9
tissue engineering   119–20
tissue inhibitor of metalloproteinases
      see TIMPs
tissue management   80, 82
topical negative pressure therapy   83,
      115–17, 189
transforming growth factors   **5**, 6
traumatic wounds   199–205
   assessment   199–201
tulle dressings   100, 110, 189, 190

undermining   75–6
urinary incontinence   131, 134,
      142, 144

vapour-permeable films   111–12
vascular endothelial growth
      factor   **5**
venous leg ulcers   151–60, 161
   aetiology   151–2
   assessment   152–4, *153*, **153**
   cleansing   155
   management   152–8
Verge Videometer   65
Visitrak   65
vitamin A   **20**
vitamin B complex   **20**
vitamin C   **20**
vitamin E   **20**
volume of wounds   66–7
vulnerability   48

Winter, George   79

wound assessment 69–75
  documentation of 74–5, 85–6
  epithelialisation 8, 73, *73*
  granulation 72–3, *73*
  infection 70–2, *70*
  necrosis 69, *69*
  slough 72, *72*

wound bed preparation 79–80, *81*
wound healing centres 230–1
wound margins 77, *78*
  advancement of 84

zinc **20**
  barrier creams 83–4

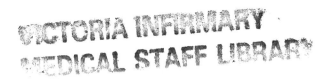